It's All About the Food

Where the American Diet Went Wrong,
Why That Matters to You, and
What You Can Do About It

by

PAT SMITH

It's All About the Food

ISBN: 978-0692567128

Trinity Books
an imprint of The Global Gospel, LLC
P.O. Box 10556
Fayetteville, Arkansas 72703

PRINTED IN THE UNITED STATES OF AMERICA

In memory of
Mitzi Price,
a dear friend lost too soon

Table of Contents

From Mount Ida to Austin

The death of my husband Gary in April of 2007 changed my life dramatically. I had retired from a long career in the telecommunications industry after a serious illness a few years prior. Gary and I moved to Mount Ida, Arkansas, at that time. We were expecting to fish in beautiful Lake Ouachita and dig in our flower garden for many more years. But we were wrong. After 46 years of marriage, I lost him. Now what was I supposed to do with the rest of my life?

Shortly after Gary died I responded to a plea in the local newspaper for volunteers to help with the Montgomery County Food Pantry—a pantry that operates under the auspices of a not-for-profit organization called Ouachita Village Inc. (or OVI). OVI is a faith-based organization not affiliated with any specific church. In a million years I would never have guessed where this simple telephone call would ultimately take me.

The woman who ran the tiny food pantry was struggling to keep it alive. She was a wonderful Christian woman with a huge heart. While she really wanted to follow her family to another town, she also didn't want the pantry to close. I was still feeling a great personal loss from my husband's death and was eager for a challenge to divert my attention. So I volunteered to take on leadership at OVI. Over three years we were able to draw many more volunteers into service. We found generous individuals, churches, and organizations to provide resources. We expanded the pantry to better meet community needs. And finally we began thinking about enlarging our programs. It was an exciting time!

While a food pantry is a crucial service for needy families, it is supposed to be a band-aid—a band-aid that, hopefully, stems the bleeding while people get their feet back on the ground. Over time, as I kept my eyes open and gathered a lot of statistics, several things became apparent. For one, many people don't even know where the ground is!

A percentage of our pantry clients at OVI are either employed in low wage jobs or in a temporary financial bind. Alice and Jacob Johnson are a good example. They were both employed and were doing fine until their daughter and her husband with three children moved in.[1] A family of two became a family of seven overnight and the income wouldn't stretch. They were embarrassed to be asking for food, but we were happy that we could help. As one would hope, the Johnsons' daughter and son-in-law eventually found employment and moved out. So the food pantry was no longer needed for the Johnsons. There have been many similar cases like theirs.

The vast majority of pantry clients are not like the Johnsons, though. Most of our clients depend on minimal Social Security support or some other sort of government aid, such as disability payments. Many have never really learned to take care of themselves. Illnesses like diabetes, obesity, and heart disease exist in almost every family and often more illness is just around the corner. The money to buy the attention of doctors and medications is frequently not available to them.

So consequently, our clients get sicker and sicker and their needs become greater and greater. More children are born into seemingly hopeless situations and the ground gets farther and farther away. We can and do throw food at the problem, but we know more is required. When I began to encounter these difficult circumstances in the lives of our clients at OVI, it made me start to ask questions: If more is required to really provide effective help, then what would "more" consist of? How might Ouachita Village Inc. help people to help themselves?

In addition to managing the food pantry, I also serve on the OVI board of directors. OVI has no paid staff, and our donations buy only food. So with the approval of our board (and on my own nickel!) I went from Montgomery County, Arkansas, to Austin, Texas, in July 2010 to find out what "more" might look like. I couldn't have predicted it at the time, but my quest would eventually lead me down trails ranging from farmer's markets to the World Wide Web. And in the process I would learn volumes on topics like the sustainable foods movement and holistic dietary nutrition. Many of the rewards would be personal, even as I set out on a mission to find out how to help people in my local community.

I chose the city of Austin because it is one of the healthiest cities in the nation. Austin is very much into the sustainable and organic growing of food, and blessed with many programs for disadvantaged people. I found not-for-profit programs in Austin helping to create gardens, service learning schools that teach vocational skills to young people, and a program that organizes and manages farmers' markets in support of small farmers and local organic food.

We like all of those programs at Ouachita Village Inc., but some serve our mission more than others. At the time of this writing OVI is working to build a Community Teaching Garden intended to teach people how to build and maintain their own gardens and to encourage neighbors to gather together in common gardens at their own initiative. While there are lots of resources and groups of people living near each other in Austin, my own community in Montgomery County, Arkansas, is a rural area with residents strewn out all over the place. The small town of Mount Ida itself has fewer than 1000 people. Consequently, a Teaching Garden makes more sense to us.

My personal favorite initiative in Austin was The Happy Kitchen nutrition and cooking class sponsored by the Sustainable Food Center. It is, in my opinion, one of Austin's shining stars. Taken with the idea of the cooking class but believing the nutritional basis to be incomplete, I set out to develop more material. That project was the beginning of what eventually became this book.

I didn't expect to get so wound up in nutrition research! I thought myself to be fairly knowledgeable before starting my research. But the more I studied the more I realized how little I actually knew. Cooking is important, but selecting the right foods is even more vital. For many of us, food selection may be the difference between being sick and being well—illness avoidance, if you will.

My investigations carried me into the thick of America's food problems. Naturally, I found out a lot about the kinds of things we hear about every day in the media. News outlets throw around a lot of nutrition and diet-related terms. They don't do a good job explaining them in layman's terms, though. With all the warnings we're bombarded with through TV and radio, magazines, and the Internet, it is hard to keep all the info straight. For example:

- The American Journal of Psychiatry reports that omega-3 deficiencies contribute to mood disorders and hurt our hearts.[2] And The Massachusetts General Hospital tells us that people deficient in vitamin D are at twice the risk of cardiovascular disease than those with normal levels of vitamin D.[3] What the heck is omega-3?

- We are told regularly that reducing fats in our diet also reduces risk of cardiovascular disease. And, in fact, in December of 2006, New York City banned trans-fats in restaurants.[4] What are trans-fats and why should we care?

- Dr. Oz, cardiac surgeon, author, and host of a daily television show focused on medical and personal health, tells us to "Read the food labels of products in your pantry and refrigerator and throw out all products that contain HFCS."[5] HFCS is high fructose corn syrup. Why should we throw these products out?

- NPR's Health Blog headline for August 10, 2011 was, "To Dodge Diabetes, Go Light on the Hot Dogs and Bacon."[6] Really!

This is only a sample of the kind of information that finds its way into our homes on a daily basis. The list can seem like an endless information overload. So when we can't handle it all, we start to dump. We tune it out just like our kids tune us out. Or we zero in on just one thing to worry about. It shouldn't be too hard to give up hot dogs if it prevents diabetes, should it? Unless, of course, a hot dog piled high with relish and mustard is your all time favorite food or perhaps the only food you think you can afford. What do you do then?

The USDA dietary guidelines are revised and revised again but some of us only know the USDA to be associated with commodity distribution (in other words, free food for low-income people). Even if we follow the USDA closely, though, it doesn't solve our problem. Every study, article, and news report on health can motivate the commercial food industry to do something to either take advantage of (or counteract) the latest news.

Sometimes that "something" is rallying the marketing people to neutralize the threat. For example, The Corn Refiners Association first tried to counteract the outcry over high fructose corn syrup by issuing (and then recalling) new commercials claiming that "whether it's corn sugar or cane sugar, your body can't tell the difference." Then they attempted to rebrand high fructose corn syrup as "corn sugar." The Food & Drug Administration (FDA) was not really taken with that idea. Now the commercials are back. Of course, all of that is beside the point when it comes to high fructose corn syrup. But the majority of us have no clue what the real point is.

The more that health is in the headlines, the more new "diets" get developed and the more books get written. That section in your local bookstore and on Amazon.com gets wider and taller every day. But we don't seem to be getting anywhere health-wise, chiefly because the average American knows almost nothing about nutrition and the operation of his or her own body. So instead we worry the most about other things. Things like our weight.

Finding the perfect diet to lose weight might be your ultimate goal, but what is the penalty for not losing weight? You look really bad in your clothes? Bummer! Unfortunately, when I started digging into material on nutrition I found countless studies describing how and why diets intended just to lose weight almost always fail in the end. Our failure to understand the problems with the "diet" concept helps to explain why two-thirds of Americans are either overweight or obese.

Through no fault of our own our heads are in the wrong place. We fail to realize that a diet is not a weight loss regimen. A diet is the way we should be eating all the time, and the consequence of poor diet is illness! Nutritionally, it isn't any one thing on that endless list of things to eat or not eat that will either save us or doom us. It is the combination of all that stuff put together, often including things that we do not even know exist. This brings us to the purpose of this book.

I support many experts, including some mentioned in this book, who are actively involved in looking for global solutions to America's healthcare issues.

But I promise you, even when they work, global solutions can take forever. So, in the meantime, we have to take responsibility individually. That is what this book is about.

It's All About the Food is <u>not</u> meant to treat illness. Doctors treat illness, and you need to see yours when you think you are not well. Nor is it a weight loss plan—although you will probably lose extra weight, especially if you fit into the two-thirds of overweight Americans I mentioned earlier.

It's All About the Food <u>is</u> meant to help you and your family members greatly reduce the risk of having one or more of the chronic and deadly diseases so common in the United States today—and to accomplish this as inexpensively as possible. The diet and nutrition focus of this book is relevant for everybody; the wealthy and middle class are not protected from poor nutrition and are often just as sick as the poor.

Starting as a novice means that research and writing this book have been a challenge for me. But the good Lord sent me to Austin, Texas! And apparently, He meant for me to finish this work in His name, for each time my resolve weakened, He propped me back up. In time I uncovered a health condition I believe He was leading me to—thanks be to God! What I discovered is that I have type 2 diabetes, and this became the turning point in my research and writing focus.

I am not and never have been overweight, which is a genetic plus for me. Just about everyone in my Dad's family was diabetic, though. I never paid any attention to this part of my family history because I believed that only fat people got diabetes, and I was never fat. I also knew that people got fat by overindulging in sugary sweets. In other words, I had no proper notion of the relationship between what I ate and the illness of diabetes. (My daughter, who is 20 years my junior, was surprised to find that I believed sugary foods made people fat. She always thought that fat made people fat! So there's more than one mistaken idea out there…)

My mother was not a baker. So growing up, I never learned to love desserts like cakes and pies that include tons of plain old refined table sugar. Naturally, I thought I was protected both from getting fat and from the illnesses (like diabetes) that I associated with obesity. Think about it. Isn't "sugar" all you hear about when it comes to gaining weight? Now I've learned that all that excess bread, crackers, chips, pasta, potatoes (as well as the flour in the cake as opposed to the sugar in the filling) are also forms of sugar. They are carbohydrates or starches, which break down into sugar in our blood. And they can be every bit as bad. Our typical American carb-heavy diet is literally making us sick.

I had what can be called a paradigm shift, a new perspective on the importance of diet and health. My attention was redirected from how to provide needy people with better food education to what causes diabetes and how diabetes is connected at the hip to other chronic diseases. As you will see in reading, the direct connection between the two and the percentage of Americans who are in danger is actually frightening. My paradigm shift ultimately made this into a different book than I thought it would be at first.

Let me offer a word of thanks: I truly appreciate the large group of concerned scientists, dieticians, nutritionists, and doctors whose expertise on diet, nutrition, and their relationship to chronic diseases has guided my reflection and writing. You will see many of their names and publications as you read ahead. What they've taught me is essential: Healthy eating can be easy, delicious, and affordable. Being well, however, should be our primary goal. As Pamela Smith has said, we should eat well in order to live well.[7] Going on diets is not a winning strategy. Instead, we need to think of our diet as how we eat in daily life. So read on and remember: It's All About the Food!

....

END NOTES

[1] While this is a real example of a client family from our food pantry at OVI, I have changed the family members' names to protect their anonymity.

[2] Gordon Parker, Neville A. Gibson, Heather Brotchie, Gabriella Heruc, Anne-Marie Rees, and Dusan Hadzi-Pavlovic, "Omega-3 Fatty Acids and Mood Disorders," The American Journal of Psychiatry 163:6 (June 2006): 969-978. Online at: http://ajp.psychiatryonline.org/article. aspx?articleID=96663 (accessed February 22, 2014).

[3] Michael J. Pencina, et al., "Lack of vitamin D may increase heart disease risk," Journal of the American Heart Association (January 8, 2008). Online at: http://www.massgeneral.org/heartcenter/news/newsarticle. aspx?id=1073 (accessed February 22, 2014).

4   MSNBC.com News Services, "New York City passes trans fat ban," Diet and Nutrition on NBCNEWS.com (December 5, 2006). Online at: http://www.nbcnews.com/id/16051436/#.UVHsVTezKSo (accessed February 22, 2014).

5   Mehmet Oz, "The Oz Diet: No more myths. No more fads. What you should eat—and why," TIME Magazine (September 12, 2011). Dr. Oz is a surgeon, author, and host of the "Dr. Oz Show," a television program focusing on medical issues and personal health.

6   Allison Aubrey, "To Dodge Diabetes, Go Light on the Hot Dogs and Bacon," NPR Health News (August 10, 2011). Online at: http://www.npr.org/blogs/health/2011/08/10/139405966/to-dodge-diabetes-go-light-on-the-hot-dogs-and-bacon (accessed February 20, 2014).

7   Pamela M. Smith, Eat Well, Live Well (Charisma House, 1992).

I Am Talking to You!

I recently watched an amazing 2012 panel discussion from BioMed Central focusing on the obesity-cancer connection. The panel was held as part of a conference on "Metabolism, Diet, and Disease" in Washington D.C. A number of experts spoke on the panel, and many others were in the audience. Some of them suggested that if obesity were eliminated in the United States today, the amount of cancer in the American population would quickly be reduced by 25% to 33%. (The remaining cancers that wouldn't be affected by a healthier, thinner population result from causes other than obesity.) So, the experts asked, should our focus be on eliminating obesity at the individual level? Or should it be on some combination of public policy together with treating the obesity and cancer medically?[1]

These are questions worth serious consideration. First, a word or two about some of the terms those panelists were using.

Public policy would be stuff like laws, rules, or regulations governing what could or couldn't be included in processed food (like trans-fats) and what could or couldn't be introduced into the environment (like chemicals). The purpose of creating policy for agriculture and food processing would be to change the kind of food we eat. By changing the kind of food we eat, we'd also change how are bodies are affected by things like additives and chemicals.

Treating, as the panel experts were using the term, would include all those medications and procedures with which we're familiar from our visits to the doctor or the hospital. It would also include any new medicines and procedures as they develop over time. Treating chronic illnesses and diseases is what health care professionals do with their suffering patients, in an attempt to halt the negative impact of the disease on the person's body. But look at what that means in the context of the obesity-cancer connection: Treating the illness amounts to finding medicines and procedures to undo the negative cancer consequences of obesity without actually doing away with the obesity.

Here is the scary part: While all the panelists agreed that the ideal fix would be to eliminate obesity, there was no faith—no faith—that the American population could be expected to change their diets and lifestyles at their own initiative. That reminds me of a quote I saw not long ago by Max Planck, Nobel Prize winner in Physics in 1918:

> A new scientific truth does not triumph by convincing its opponents and making them see the light, but rather because its opponents die and a new generation grows up that is familiar with it.[2]

Ouch. A quote like that makes me truly respect the amazing group of advocates in the area of food and nutrition who are working tirelessly everyday to influence both public policy and personal behavior. It's hard work and progress is measured slowly. Bad habits are always hard to break. That's as true of bad food habits as it is of drug and alcohol abuse.

I want to make sure that we adapt to the new information that is now available to us in a way that Dr. Planck didn't think many people could. That's why I am willing to take the direct approach. That's why I am talking to you.

Are you personally willing to leave it to public policy or politics to decide what you should eat? It took public policy influenced by politics over 20 years to publically expose trans-fats as bad for us while we were being exposed to the consequences every single day of that time. Are you really willing to depend on medical treatments to delay the inevitable? Are you satisfied to be one of the "opponents" of new scientific findings who remain smug in their opinions even while they are dying off?

If not, then this book may change your life.

END NOTES

[1]   "Panel discussion from 'Metabolism Diet and Disease' conference held in Washington DC, May 29-31, 2012," BioMed Central: The Open Access Publisher [www.biomedcentral.com] (May 2012). Online at: http://www.biomedcentral.com/series/metabolismdietanddisease (accessed November 8, 2014).

[2]   Entry for "Max Planck," Wikiquote [http://en.wikiquote.org/]. Online at: http://en.wikiquote.org/w/index.php?title=Max_Planck&oldid=1819023 (accessed November 8, 2014).

CHAPTER TWO

The American Diet and Overweight Gorillas

This unfortunate report about a new resident in the London Zoo appeared in the spring of 2010:

> Yeboah, the 12-year-old western lowland gorilla brought over to London Zoo in November from La Boissière du Doré zoo in France … died suddenly last Thursday, 25th March. He'd earlier recorded high blood sugar levels, so diabetes is suspected but not confirmed.[1]

Yeboah was actually the second male gorilla to die at the London Zoo's Gorilla Kingdom, which opened in 2007. Another gorilla named Bobby died at age 25 in December of 2008. Bobby is believed to have had a heart attack. In captivity, the life expectancy of this species of gorilla is 35 to 45 years.

Yet Bobby and Yeboah are not the only gorillas that have died unexpectedly in recent years. It is something of an epidemic. Gorillas have died untimely deaths in many zoos, primarily from progressive heart ailments. Whatever could be causing it? In 2006, a number of zoos banded together looking for answers. After extensive research the Cleveland Zoo took two important steps. First, they placed two gorillas that were already diagnosed with heart disease on typical human medications. Secondly, they stopped feeding them a steady diet of processed starch/sugar biscuits and substituted instead wheelbarrows full of greens, endive, green beans, and hay, along with fruit—a diet closer to their diet in the wild with higher fiber and simple, non-starchy sugar.

So what was the outcome? Well, it isn't over yet but after more than a year on their new diet, the two gorillas had lost about 65 pounds apiece while consuming twice the calories, getting them close to the weight of their counterparts in the wild.[2] The next step, they say, is exercising the gorillas in zoos.

Why, you may ask, am I telling you this? We aren't gorillas, you and I (although our DNA is close!). So what does the health of gorillas have to do with the health of human beings?

First, take note. We humans have been told for some time that our heart disease is the result of the consumption of cholesterol and saturated fat associated with animal protein. Well—surprise, surprise—gorillas do not eat much animal protein. They are essentially herbivores whose protein consumption consists largely of insects, termites, and such. How the heck are they getting heart disease?

Here is how. The food being provided to the gorillas at many zoos consists of the very same processed starch and sugar that most Americans (and lots of other folks across the world) consume in large quantities every single day of our lives. Did you notice that Yeboah, the first gorilla in the London Zoo article, had high blood sugar suspected to indicate diabetes? We humans and the gorillas are eating the same food and getting the same diseases.

An edition of the Austin Statesman newspaper in November 2010 featured the following headline: "Starved for information? Well, there's nothing happy about obesity."[3] The article was about McDonald's Happy Meals with included toys. In it, the reporter concluded, "And this is where a child's desire for a fun treat, a parent's desire to cheaply feed and simultaneously entertain their kids, and a profound ignorance of the basic tenets of nutrition intersect to fuel the obesity epidemic in this country."[4]

That reporter was right on target. Look around in your community. Not only are the gorillas overweight, but two-thirds of your neighbors and friends are overweight as well. Half of them are obese—all overfed and many undernourished. And that's not all there is to it. In seeming lockstep, levels of type 2 diabetes continue to rise. Is that a fluke? Did the stars line up just right or is there a connection here?

For years we have heard how important it is to cut back on cholesterol and avoid saturated fat, the thick stuff that runs through beef, coats the chicken, and makes up the largest percentage of our (very favorite) bacon. These two, the experts said, are clogging our arteries. We can fix that, they insisted, by cutting back on cholesterol and saturated animal fat. Were they right?

Over the last 40 years Americans have been cutting back on cholesterol and saturated animal fats. Less beef, more chicken, cut off that skin and trim off that fat. And what did we get for that reduction? According to the EPA the frequency rate of cardiovascular disease (CVD) has remained essentially constant (unchanged) for the last 10 years.[5] What has changed, however, is the death rate and cost, both in dollars and pain. Americans are living longer with CVD according to the American Heart Association's Heart Disease and Stroke Statistics reports for 2010[6] and 2012,[7] an accomplishment seemingly made possible by a 22% increase in inpatient operations and procedures. We spend a lot of money on cardiovascular disease treatment and medicine. We can make people live longer but we can't seem to reduce the level of sickness.

So heart and circulatory disease, obesity, and diabetes are rampant disorders in America, and the food we eat is playing a major role in these conditions. This does not have to be! The zookeepers have a leg up on this because they are able to control the amount and kind of food being fed to the gorillas. In the case of humans, we have free choice. But good choices require a level of knowledge and a willingness to change that many of us don't seem to have.

It really boils down to a simple question: What is your risk tolerance? Every year my financial planner asks me that question again. The market will always go up and down, he reminds me, so how fearful am I of losing a percentage of my investments? More of my savings is now sitting in bonds and money market accounts where they don't make much money but are relatively safe from loss. My risk tolerance has changed over the years.

Consider the risks attached to stuff like snow skiing, parasailing, motorcycle racing without a helmet, driving on snow or icy streets, breaking the speed limit, driving without a license or insurance, stealing, buying a house or a car, walking alone in a park at night, having that one last child after the doctor warns you against it, and boating without a life jacket. Sometimes we know immediately our risk tolerance based on the condition of our stomach when we think about it. This is called fear. But some of us have no fear. Some of us ignore odds and consequences and focus only on the potential joy of the experience. Can't you just feel the wind blowing through your hair? And besides, it's hot inside that motorcycle helmet. Yeah, a wreck might splatter you all over the road. But bad stuff happens to other people, not you. Right?

My dad could not swim. Despite that, he often went frog gigging in a boat with my uncle at night with absolutely no thought of a life jacket! He was, to say the least, very risk tolerant. My mother, who also could not swim, would not go near a body of water larger than the bathtub. Does it surprise you that my sister and I were in swimming classes before we even went to school?

Some risks seem almost unavoidable. You are broke and have to go to work. So although you don't have insurance for your car and your license is suspended for that very reason, you still have to go to work. Soooooo. You are terrified of fire but will rush into a burning building to save a child. High risk tolerance under the circumstances. Or, as they say, you do what you gotta do. Just because some risks are unavoidable, though, that doesn't mean all of them have to be.

This brings us back to health and food. Are you paying all your attention to the joy of eating and not considering the consequences of your food choices? In the pages that follow, you are going to learn about things you should and should not eat. But you and you alone can decide your risk tolerance. In order for you to determine that for yourself, you need to know the consequences of your choices. My goal is to help you make an informed decision.

END NOTES

[1]   Robert Hanks, "Zoo news: dead gorilla," Zoo in the head blog (April 2, 2010). Online at: http://roberthanks.typepad.com/zoo_in_the_head/2010/04/zoo-news-dead-gorilla.html (accessed February 22, 2014).

[2]   Case Western Reserve University, "Gorillas go green: Apes shed pounds while doubling calories on leafy diet, researcher finds," Science Daily. Online at: www.sciencedaily.com/releases/2011/02/110217091130.htm (accessed November 20, 2014).

[3]   Esther J. Cepeda, "Starved for information? Well, there's nothing happy about obesity," Austin (Texas) Statesman (November 13, 2010).

[4]   Ibid. Italics added.

[5]   Donald Lloyd-Jones, et al., "Executive Summary: Heart Disease and Stroke Statistics—2010 Update: A Report from the American Heart Association," Circulation 121:7 (February 2010): 948-954. Online at: http://circ.ahajournals.org/content/121/7/e46.full.pdf (accessed November 20, 2014).

[6]   Ibid.

[7]   Véronique L. Roger, et al., "Heart Disease and Stroke Statistics—2012 Update: A Report from the American Heart Association," Circulation 125:1 (January 2012): e2. Online at: http://circ.ahajournals.org/content/early/2011/12/15/CIR.0b013e31823ac046.full.pdf (accessed February 25, 2014).

CHAPTER THREE

How Your Body Works: A Short Description

Everything absorbed by our body from the environment is processed by our body. Everything we put in our mouths, breathe in through our noses, touch with our skin is broken down and converted by the body into multiple elements needed for us to remain healthy. All of those elements interact with each other in ways so complex that many, if not most, are not fully understood.

The conversion process called metabolism always leaves a residue inside of us. This is left-over stuff that, if not dealt with, can be deadly. But our amazing bodily systems are designed to take care of that. Some substances, like nitrites and fructose and even trans-fats (as examples of things constantly in the nutrition limelight) occur naturally in almost all animal and plant food. When we eat the natural food that contains them, our systems get the value from the food, sweep aside the trash, and then discard it. Everything we need to gain the value and deal with the residue is included in our food. But when those substances are extracted or chemically created and inserted into processed foods, the outcome can be different.

So at a grand level, many of the problems occurring in our health are caused by mankind's attempts to artificially reproduce things that occur naturally in nature and then use them for our unique purposes. The food and drug industries have a big motivation to develop, test, and sell the consumer products that result from this kind of lab research and experimentation. Three factors help to explain how this is the case:

The Profit Factor

Corporations exist to provide goods and services to the public for a profit. (No big surprise there.) Profit for a company increases when that company can get its product in your hands as cheaply as possible. In the food industry, this has resulted in these two trends:

- Growing the food, both animal and plant, in unnatural ways in order to minimize expense, all the while creating ever growing new lines of "products."

- Encouraging the consumption of "created" food products through effective advertising while minimizing the expense of getting them to your table through lower cost-of-production.

The Transportation Factor

Consumer desire to have the full range of food products at all times of the year has led to the practice of harvesting, packaging, or even "creating" foods in one place like, say, California and moving it to another place like Arkansas without spoiling. Think of this as the "Oranges in December" rule.

The Lifestyle Accommodation Factor

Because the American public wants to eat what it wants, when it wants, and in the amount that it wants, there are serious health consequences to deal with. Drug companies therefore move to treat conditions caused, in many cases, by what the first two factors have allowed to happen. This requires a whole new avenue of "products" mostly related to medicine rather than food.

The result is that we are eating "food" that includes substances different from what our body was designed to handle. Ingesting these substances over the long term will inevitably make us sick. Then we end up taking "medications" to counteract the ill effects of those artificially processed foods.

Our bodies were made to eat and digest natural foods that occur in our world— both animals and plants. What our bodies have trouble with is food that has been transformed by additives and chemicals that wouldn't naturally occur in the foods that now contain them. Put gasoline in your car, and it will run fine. But put lemonade in the gas tank, and the car will break down pretty quickly!

With the vast changes in the American diet over the past hundred years, we've begun putting things in our gas tanks that were never meant to be there. The results? Predictable, unfortunately. Now let's explore in fairly simple terms how all this happened and what the major consequences have been.

CHAPTER FOUR

The Last
100 Years

A number of changes in the American lifestyle have occurred over the last 100 or so years, some good and some not-so-good. A not-so-good change is that the family farm with its natural, healthy supply of meat and vegetables has largely disappeared. It has been replaced by commercial animal feedlots, industrial truck farms, processed food manufacturers, and large grocery stores. If you don't grow your own food, you have to get it somewhere.

When I was a kid, my grandma and grandpa lived on what might today be called a mini-farm. The garden was huge and the vegetables we ate came from that garden. The hogs (the sausage from which was mixed in a big iron kettle in the yard), chickens (whose necks got wrung right before my eyes so we could have chicken for Sunday dinner), and eggs all came from the same farm. My grandma canned or dried everything—including beef when the occasional cow was butchered. (My cousin assures me that beef from a jar is disgusting. I'm happy to say I never tried it.) They had a real "ice box." Many of you in my age group probably have equally vivid memories of locally grown food from your own childhood.

As they grew older, grandma and grandpa couldn't manage all of that. Like most of us today, they began eating the stuff from the store. "Fresh" was no longer the name of the game. In time their health, particularly my grandpa's, suffered. They didn't realize it at the time, but their old fashioned way of raising and harvesting their own food had directly contributed to their longevity. When they "went with the times" out of convenience and old age, the processed items on the shelf of the local grocery store did them no favors.

From Farm to Feedlot

Commercial feedlots changed the food supply for farm animals from the pasture grass of my grandpa's farm to starchy, grain based food—largely corn. This wasn't and isn't good for the cows. Check out how Dr. Don Montgomery, a veterinary scholar at the University of Wyoming, describes the effects of this change:

> From a nutritional perspective, these animals [i.e., cattle] are pushed to the maximum using concentrated, high carbohydrate-based rations to effect efficient feed conversion and marketing within a customary time frame. Although effective from an economic standpoint, such rations can contribute to or cause serious digestive disturbances...[1]

Did you catch that? The "carbohydrate-based rations" (or grain) make the cows fat as fast as possible so they can be delivered to the market as quickly as possible. The "customary time frame" that Dr. Montgomery mentions is just a reference to the rush-to-market approach of the commercial food industry that puts the bare economics of the process above all else.

Why does that matter? Well, the same thing happens to the cattle that happened to those gorillas in the London Zoo. Beyond getting fat quickly, they also get sick. Cows get sick primarily because a cow's digestive system is designed for grass, not for grain. (That's why Dr. Montgomery's description refers to certain "digestive disturbances.") The feedlot operators anticipate the cows' illness and give them (along with pigs and chickens in industrial farm environments) ongoing antibiotics to promote weight gain, since the "carbohydrate-based rations" that make up their food aren't enough on their own.

Antibiotics aren't just used to combat the effects of the feeding practices, though. The drugs also help to counter the fact that their living conditions are so unsanitary. Cattle are packed together shoulder-to-shoulder, standing in their own manure. Each cow in a feedlot is susceptible to whatever illness any one of the others gets. (Just as when one child in a daycare center gets sick you can bet the rest will catch it!) So sick cows are then given even more antibiotics—in fact, a remarkable 80% of all the antibiotics used in the United States are given to livestock animals.[2] Cows in a feedlot will never be healthy in any real sense, but they're slaughtered before they can die of the dismal conditions they live in. And then we eat them. (Isn't that a pleasant thought!)

Not only is this not good for the cows, it also isn't good for those of us who eat the cows. The more antibiotics are given, the more that germs will become resistant to them. This is a big, big issue these days for human health in hospitals where drug-resistant bacteria make fighting infection more difficult everyday. But when it comes to nutrition, the impact of those "carbohydrate-based rations" on the meat is the most important concern. So what does all that grain do to the beef that ends up going to your local grocery store?

Beef (and other meats) contain a variety of nutrients critical to our bodies. Among those nutrients are omega-6 and omega-3 fatty acids found in the animal fat. The proper balance of these two substances will nurture the body's immune system. A relatively even balance of omega-6 to omega-3 fatty acids in pasture-fed beef changes to something like a 30:1 ratio or more (depending on whom you ask) in grain-fed beef. The ratio of omega-6 to omega-3 gets all out of whack, in other words. And that is <u>way</u> too much omega-6 for those of us who end up eating the beef.

The reason all this happens is relatively simple. It is related to the cows' diet. Cattle get all that extra omega-6 from the corn they are fed—which is naturally high in omega-6 fatty acid. Too much omega-6 contributes to chronic low-grade inflammation in the body of the human eating the meat. The relationship of omega-6 fatty acid to low-grade inflammation in people is a topic we'll have much more to say about later. For now just make note of the word "inflammation." You're going to hear it a lot!

The Rise of the Processed Food Era

One hundred years ago our family farms were fertilized with the manure conveniently delivered by cattle that lived on the farm and not by the chemical fertilizers commonly used today. Just like my grandma, our ancestors went into their gardens, picked the vegetables, took them to the kitchen, and cooked and ate them. The shelves of our root cellars were lined with canned and dried foods to carry us through the winter. The small farms and gardens of that time provided their fare seasonally. That means, among other things, that we grew grains like wheat and corn when they were in season. The food supply over the year varied but was balanced. We worked really hard maintaining that food supply: we ground our own grain and made our own bread, milked our own cows and churned our own butter.

When family farms were replaced by industrial truck farms, three critical changes occurred. First, chemical fertilizers came into use, then pesticides for those pesky insects, and finally herbicides to hold down the weeds. Eventually the farmland soil was damaged and the produce itself was contaminated. That was bad news for us, because those chemical contaminants eventually found their way into our bodies. Chemical contamination then began to contribute both to environmental pollutants and low-grade inflammation in our bodies. It made us sick and it made our environment sick as well.

Secondly, the short trip from the field to the kitchen became a long truck, train, or boat ride across the country. Or even across the world. As food ages in a shipping container (as well as on the grocery store shelf), it deteriorates. That makes fewer nutrients available to the person who eats the food. Fewer nutrients in the food results in less nutritious food overall.

Thirdly and lastly, the federal government responded to the Great Depression of the 1930s with subsidies and programs to prop up grain farmers. The farmers and their suppliers used the subsidies to figure out how to keep grain available year around. Unlike cauliflower or peppers or other fresh vegetables, properly dried grain (such as wheat or corn) can be stored for a very long time. With a limitless supply of grain, commercial food processors were then positioned to make grain and grain-based products available 24 hours a day, 7 days a week. The amount of farmland committed to grain production naturally grew by leaps and bounds—and was aided by the technological changes that were ongoing at the same time and which replaced farm labor with farm machinery. This was the beginning of the Processed Food Era, which has seen grain consumption in the American diet simply skyrocket.[3] Just like eating grain-fed beef, eating large quantities of grain directly results in an out-of-whack omega-6 fatty acid buildup. This, too, has caused damage to our bodies.

For many Americans, the absence of good fresh garden produce was seen as no big deal at the time because processed food (that stuff in boxes, cans, and jars on the grocery store shelves) soon replaced fresh foods. Just like it did at my grandma's house. In fact, it was easier to buy your groceries at the local Piggly Wiggly than it was to raise the food yourself! The end result? Now

Americans eat 31% more processed food than they do fresh food.[4] In fact, according to food writer Melanie Warner, about 70% of our calories come from processed food.[5] The vast majority of that processed food has loads of chemical additives and preservatives. It usually contains added sugar of some sort. Practically all of it is either grain-based (like bread and pasta) or includes grain oils. The kind of agriculture it takes to produce that grain does damage to both you and the land. We've come a long way from grandpa's farm.

Partially Hydrogenated Grain Oils…in Everything

Wait—grain oils? Did you say grain oils?? What the heck are these? As it turns out, the oil that is extracted from grains like soybeans and corn play a huge role in the processed food story.

All fat, both animal and vegetable, contains some mixture of polyunsaturated, monounsaturated, and saturated fats. But vegetable oils made from grain are primarily polyunsaturated and make an even bigger contribution to inflammation in the human body than the grain-fed cattle mentioned earlier. Why, you ask? In proper proportions, polyunsaturated fats are not bad. In fact, omega-6 and its partner omega-3 fatty acids are polyunsaturated and they are both essential nutritional elements for our bodies. But because the oils extracted from grain are concentrated, they are not just high but extremely high in omega-6 fatty acid. They are the oil of choice in processed foods (and we eat a lot more processed foods than we eat beef). Grain-based oils such as corn oil, often referred to simply as vegetable oil, have also become a stand-by in most American kitchens.[6]

One of the central issues in processed foods is shelf life. Many, if not most, processed foods include oil. In the old days, saturated fat from animals and saturated vegetable oils like coconut and palm were the oils of choice because those oils stay solid and stable without spoiling. But in 1911, Crisco shortening became the first manufactured food product to include partially hydrogenated oil.[7] This is a type of vegetable oil that has been chemically modified so it will act saturated, meaning that it won't turn to liquid at room temperature or quickly spoil. In time we found partially hydrogenated oils in practically all processed foods. Partially hydrogenated oil produces trans-fats, which we now know are very bad for us.

The corn oil on the shelf at the grocery isn't hydrogenated. However, except when grain oil is expeller pressed (which isn't often because it is more expensive), the process of extracting the oil from the corn occurs at a high temperature and includes chemicals which damage the oil and neutralize the antioxidants that protect the oil from oxidation. The resulting oil is susceptible to heat, light, and oxygen. When exposed to air and heat too long as in frying or just sitting on your pantry shelf, it will oxidize and become rancid very quickly. Oxidized, rancid oils also become trans-fats.

The absence of fresh vegetables in our diet deprives our bodies of a world of antioxidants and anti-inflammatories (vitamins, phytonutrients, etc.). That's the stuff that is the first and last line of defense against chronic bodily inflammation and disease. And the persistent presence of grain oil in our diet makes those deficiencies an even bigger problem.

As I said before, we've come a long way from grandpa's farm. In the grand scheme of things, commercial food processing has been, perhaps, the very worst change of the last few decades. The effects of it crept up on us while we weren't looking. Beyond the overabundance of omega-6 in grain and grain oils that can lead to problems for people whose diets are mostly grain-based, food processing removes basic nutrients from the food. It introduces a world of chemical additives and preservatives. And it's produced with very unhealthy chemically modified fats and sugars like partially hydrogenated vegetable oils (trans-fats) and high fructose corn syrup.

While all of these changes to food production and the American diet were going on, cardiovascular disease started skyrocketing in the U.S. population. So with the encouragement of the United States Department of Agriculture (USDA) and the American Heart Association (AHA), the food industry began pushing for changes in public policy that it claimed would make us healthier: reducing cholesterol consumption, reducing fat in milk and other dairy products (as well as in processed foods), adding sugar or sugar substitutes in place of the fats, and using the above mentioned vegetable oils to replace animal fats for cooking. These were all supposed to be good changes, but they all missed the point about what really causes us harm.

A lot has changed over 100 years. And so we are sick.

Coda: The Obesity Epidemic

Here's some amazing information from the Center for Sustainable Systems at the University of Michigan: Between 1970 and 2009 the average American's daily calorie intake increased from 2169 to 2594 calories.[8] That is almost a 20% increase in calories every single day.

Generally speaking, an extra 500 calories per day is supposed to buy you one extra pound per week, 52 pounds per year. As we will learn later, the number of calories is actually less important than the source of those calories. Here's the rub: that calorie increase over the past 40 years came primarily from grains, fats, and sugar—most of which are consumed in the form of nutrient-poor refined, processed foods. These were not calories from vegetables; the consumption of vegetables in the population has remained at a consistently low level.

So with that level of increasing calorie consumption, can we be surprised that over a third of Americans are overweight and another third are obese? Here's the disheartening statistic on my own home state of Arkansas: "Fifteen years ago, Arkansas had a combined obesity and overweight rate of 51.8 percent. Ten years ago, it was 57.9 percent. Now, the combined rate is 66.5 percent ... [and] 20.4 percent of children and adolescents in Arkansas [aged 10-17] are considered obese."[9] Those statistics are frightening.

With a more overweight population, we will see a sharp increase in chronic diseases related to obesity and unhealthy eating. Take diabetes as an example. Not only is type 2 diabetes increasing across the U.S. population, but according to a recent study by the American Diabetes Association, the size of the diabetes population and the related costs in the United States are also "expected to at least double in the next 25 years."[10]

We are managing to keep people with cardiovascular disease alive longer but not without cost. Americans have more chronic diseases, take more medicines, and spend more for medical treatment than any other country in the world. Persistent inflammation in our bodies caused by our lifestyle and food choices is the major contributor. All in all, we have created quite a mess for ourselves.

END NOTES

[1]   Don Montgomery, DVM, PhD, "Feedlot Diseases of Cattle and Sheep,"
      University of Wyoming course lecture (orig., February 23, 2006; updated
      August 11, 2010). Online at: http://www.uwyo.edu/vetsci/undergraduates/
      courses/patb_4110/2009_lectures/15_feedlot/html/class_notes.htm
      (accessed July 23, 2014).

[2]   As reported in the New York Times on April 15, 2012, "Last Wednesday, the
      Food and Drug Administration issued new regulatory guidelines, as part of
      an effort to get drug companies, animal producers and veterinarians to rein
      in indiscriminate use of antibiotics that are important for treating humans.
      There is a lot of reining in to do — about 80 percent of all antibiotics sold in
      the United States are used in animals, the vast majority to promote rapid
      weight gain, not to treat sick animals" (from "Antibiotics Off the Farm,"
      New York Times editorial [April 15, 2012]). Online at: http://www.nytimes.
      com/2012/04/16/opinion/antibiotics-off-the-farm.html (accessed February
      25, 2014).

[3]   The shifts in the American diet towards extremely high levels of grain
      consumption through a dizzying variety of processed foods would contribute
      mightily to a sharp increase in omega-6 fatty acid in the average person,
      which leads to chronic inflammation in the body (There's that word again—
      inflammation).

[4]   Tom Laskawy, "Americans eat more processed food than, well, anyone," Grist
      Magazine (April 8, 2010). Online at: http://grist.org/article/americans-eat-
      more-processed-food-than-well-anyone/ (accessed February 27, 2014).

[5]   Melanie Warner, Pandora's Lunchbox: How Processed Food Took Over the
      American Meal (New York: Scribner, 2013).

[6]   According to a 2006 report by the Corn Refiner's Association, "Corn oil is
      now the second leading vegetable oil produced in the United States, second
      in importance only to soybean oil. Domestic corn oil production was 2.5
      billion pounds in 2004[.]" See Corn Refiner's Association, Corn Oil, 5th
      edition (Washington, DC, 2006), 19. Available online at: http://www.corn.org/
      wp-content/uploads/2009/12/CornOil.pdf (accessed October 14, 2014).

7   American Heart Association, "A History of Trans Fat," AHA Website [www.heart.org] (August, 2010). Online at: http://www.heart.org/ HEARTORG/GettingHealthy/FatsAndOils/Fats101/A-History-of-Trans-Fat_ UCM_301463_Article.jsp#.TydmMYEU7To (accessed February 20, 2014).

8   "US Environmental Footprint Factsheet," Center for Sustainable Systems at the University of Michigan (October 2014). Online at: http://css.snre.umich. edu/css_doc/CSS08-08.pdf (accessed November 12, 2014).

9   New Report: Arkansas is Ninth Most Obese State in the Nation," Report from the Trust for America's Health Organization (July 7, 2011). Online at: http://healthyamericans.org/reports/obesity2011/release.php?stateid=AR (accessed February 25, 2014).

10 Elbert S. Huang, et al., "Projecting the Future Diabetes Population Size and Related Costs for the U.S.," Diabetes Care 32:12 (December 2009): 22225-22229. Online at: http://care.diabetesjournals.org/content/32/12/2225.full. pdf (accessed November 14, 2014). Diabetes Care is the journal of the American Diabetes Association.

CHAPTER FIVE

The Almost Perfect Diet

— THE SHORT VERSION —

I asked my friend Ann to read an early draft of the book you now hold in your hands. She gave me many helpful suggestions! One of the best ones was that I should "cut to the chase" and just tell her what she needs to do. There's a lot of important material in the story I have to tell. But for those of you who (like Ann) want the short version right away, here it is: The Almost Perfect Diet.

As we have seen, for most Americans inflammation is largely the result of inflicting damage on ourselves through our diet or lifestyle. Diminish that damage by taking these steps:

- Eliminate or at least minimize the consumption of refined, processed foods and food products, including those with preservatives and additives. That is the stuff in sacks, bags, jars, boxes, and other kinds of packages sitting on the shelves in the middle of the grocery store and in the bakery. Read the label. And replace that boxed, packaged, processed stuff with fresh foods whenever possible.

  - If you must use processed foods, make sure that any oil included is either extra virgin olive oil (EVOO) or canola oil.

  - Particularly avoid processed foods that contain hydrogenated or partially hydrogenated oil of any kind. These will inevitably be trans-fats.

- Keep foods containing refined sugar and/or high fructose corn syrup to an absolute minimum. Most people don't eat refined sugar by the spoonful (except maybe in coffee) and I have personally never seen a container of high fructose corn syrup (HFCS). Instead we most often get these sugars in the processed foods mentioned above. Work hard to find sweet recipes for your own kitchen that include little or no refined sugar. This is possible. It takes a little work on the front end, but once you find a few recipes that you like they can become your "go to" desserts.

- Limit starch (grain and potato) consumption to two servings per meal, six servings per day unless you are diabetic or pre-diabetic. Then the limit may be three or even less. Attend to serving sizes, and don't overdo it.

- If you eat processed grain, make sure it is whole grain and not refined.

- Do not eat carbohydrate starches (beans, potatoes, and particularly grain) and sugars alone. Combine them with some form of protein, fat, and fiber.

- Make extra virgin olive oil (and possibly canola oil) your cooking oil of choice. Make EVOO your salad oil of choice. Coconut oil can be used for many purposes.

- Eat lots and lots of vegetables and 2-3 servings of fruit per day. Get those veggies fresh! Have fun finding your closest farmer's market and become a regular customer. And as much as possible, make fruit your sweet of choice (rather than sugary processed junk).

- Limit meat to one serving (or less) per day.

- When possible, eat pasture raised/free range or wild caught meat as well as wild caught cold water fish (canned, fresh, or frozen). These will provide both your vitamin B12 and omega-3 requirements. Flax and chia seed are also alternative plant-based sources for omega-3.

- Beans (which are also a starch), wild caught fresh water fish, nuts, eggs, and milk products including cheese are also legitimate and desirable meat substitutes for part of your protein requirement. Remember that vegetables also include a small amount of protein.

- Make commercially processed meats such as hotdogs, salami, sausages, deli meat, etc. containing chemical preservative nitrites a much smaller portion of your overall meat consumption.

- Minimize exposure to chemical fertilizers, pesticides, and unnecessary drugs. This means the ideal vegetables and fruit would be organic or at least grown locally. All vegetables should be washed thoroughly before eating but non-organic vegetables will need extra attention. Just remember, the most important thing to do is eat fruits and vegetables—organic or not.

- Give up soft drinks. If you like the bubbles, try carbonated water.

- And don't smoke.

Those are the rules for my almost perfect diet. (Ok, smoking has nothing to do with diet but I thought it was too important to leave out for reasons I will provide later.)

Now, having seen the short version, I am anticipating your reactions. "Avoid" and "eliminate" are such a strong words, don't you think? Did I really have to use words like that? I have suggested you change your diet and that of your children, but most people don't like to change. It's a big deal. I won't pretend otherwise. The majority of us spend our lives—whether that is 71 years in my case or 2 years in the case of my great granddaughter—learning to like what we eat. Early on, we learn to take what our parents give us without asking too many questions. Later, we make our own choices. We may understand at the "head level" why what we eat isn't right or why smoking isn't good for us. But often that doesn't stop us from consuming whatever tastes good. It's that risk tolerance thing.

I was in a retail store recently and overheard a clerk in conversation with her co-worker. "I don't like water," she said as she packaged my purchase. "I just can't drink it. I drink Coke." Fortunately she was looking at my package and not my face, as I am sure I grimaced. How does one reach the point that she doesn't "like" something as neutral as water? If nothing else, this highlights the reluctance to change that many us have. We develop habits and then stick with them—whether they're healthy or not!

Maybe your attitude goes something like this: Abandoning white bread or, in my case, those yummy yeast rolls is simply out of the question. You didn't grow up eating asparagus or spinach or cauliflower and you don't want to start now. You need meat, you say, at every meal because you have always had meat at every meal. You don't like seafood. Olive oil costs too much. And you don't like whole grain cereals; you like the kind with interesting shapes, well-fortified with sugar in and on it. When you are feeling low or a little stressed, a bag of Cheetos or tortilla chips hits the spot. You have a serious sweet tooth and if you can't have things that taste good, then what's the point? Maybe you just aren't convinced that changing your diet is important enough.

If you are like me, you want reasons. If you tell me what I ought to do, then I want to know why! The more unattractive the change, the more detail I want in the explanation. The next few sections of the book will provide that detail in increasing depth. But as I think you'll see, the dietary devil is in the details. Think about this: the longer you wait to take charge of your own health, the harder it will be—and the greater the risk you have for something major going wrong. At some point, who knows where, you will make a decision to either change your diet or take your chances. How is your risk tolerance?

CHAPTER SIX

Inflammation

Inflammation can occur anywhere in the body, for a variety of reasons. In this book we are focusing on inflammation in a very specific context: the persistent inflammatory levels currently widespread in many Americans' collective blood vessels.

Inflammation is an unavoidable and, in fact, desirable byproduct of bodily processes. It happens as a result of our immune system in action. The immune system, yours and mine, defends our bodies against infection and injury. To some degree, it is even meant to protect you from yourself.   Sometimes an injury is obvious, like a broken leg or a sore throat. Last week in a fit of carelessness, I hung a fishhook in my thumb. In short order my immune system kicked into action and my thumb became hot and red. That's a good example of inflammation protecting me from me! Sometimes we can't see the inflammation, though, when an injury is more complex. Sometimes the damage is hiding out inside the body, and the symptoms are even scarier—arthritis pain, a heart attack or stroke, or crumbling bones.

There are many sources of inflammation, like free radicals for example. These are not only a source but also a result of inflammation. Just being alive—breathing, digesting food, building/replacing body cells, exercising, exposure to environmental contaminants like weed killer and fertilizer, the residue of high blood sugar, smoking—creates alien-sounding things called free radicals in your body. Free radicals are the garbage left over from ongoing cell metabolism and they can do a lot of damage. The body is designed to compensate for the free radicals created by breathing, digesting food, exercise, and building/replacing body cells. But it struggles to handle all the new substances introduced into our diets through both crops and livestock in the last 100 years.

As with all damage, the body's first response to free radicals is inflammation. Omega-6 fatty acid lights the fire and omega-3 drags out the hose. If the immune system can't finish the job and make the inflammation go away, then inflammation becomes chronic and goes on to produce lots more free radicals. These extra free radicals will, in turn, create more inflammation. Multiply that by a jillion and you have a heck of a chain reaction. Along with omega-3, the cleanup crew to stop free radicals includes the antioxidants mentioned earlier. Antioxidants are thus a crucial part of our immune system and help to defuse inflammation.

Here is how it is supposed to work: Some sort of damage is done, the immune system kicks into gear, white blood cells release chemicals that cause inflammation, the battle begins, the injury is healed, and the inflammation disappears. Life is good. The bad news happens when inflammation goes on and on and things never get back to "normal." If your immune system is compromised or your lifestyle is simply too unhealthy, you can develop chronic inflammation to a degree that the consequences are severe.

Dr. Andrew Weil, creator of The Anti-inflammatory Diet, sums it up nicely in a recent article. He writes:

> Inflammation is the cornerstone of the body's healing response. It is the process by which the immune system delivers more nourishment and more defensive activity to an area that is injured or under attack. But inflammation is so powerful and so potentially destructive that it must stay where it is supposed to be and end when it is supposed to end; otherwise it damages the body and causes disease.[1]

That means that inflammation is good, even vital, when you've been injured or when you're sick. But what if your body seems always to be sick due to the diet and lifestyle you've adopted? That's when inflammation becomes chronic and damaging.

In fact, it is exactly through a certain diet and lifestyle that many Americans have become victims of chronic inflammation. If this describes you, then you should realize that you may not even have consciously chosen the path you are now on. You just ate what everybody else was eating! That means you are a product of our food-sick culture. It also means that it's up to you to do something about it from here on out.

If you want the dietary dilemma in a nutshell, here's a summary of what we have done to ourselves:

- Limited and in some cases incapacitated our immune systems by:

    - Eating too much omega-6 fatty acids in grain-fed animals as well as vegetable oils and processed food found on the grocery shelves, too often in the form of trans-fats, and not eating enough foods containing omega-3 fatty acids to balance the omega-6.

    - Failing to eat a balanced diet including fruits and vegetables, thereby depriving the body of much-needed vitamins, antioxidants, and other vital nutrients as well as fiber.

- Expanded the load on our immune systems through:

    - Eating commercially processed, refined foods and food "products" that are reduced or absent of nutrition, contain trans-fats, produce excess levels of blood sugar/insulin in the blood, and make you fat. Excess body fat, all by itself, also generates body acid and inflammation.

    - Allergic reactions. Three of the top eight allergens in this country are dairy, wheat, and soy.[2] One or more of these three will be found in almost every commercially processed food. Gluten sensitivity and intolerance as well as Celiac disease are all associated with wheat as well as barley, rye, and sometimes oats. Allergic reactions are forms of inflammation.

    - The damage done to our environment and our animal and plant food sources by toxins, chemical fertilizers, pesticides, hormones and antibiotics, and (potentially) genetically modified food sources.

    - Smoking and drug usage.

This, my friends, is not a trick. Consider yourself. Did you know about inflammation before reading this book? Do any or all of the sources of inflammation described above apply to you? The potential consequences of that inflammation include some downright deadly stuff.

Here are some of the diseases and chronic conditions linked to inflammation:

- Diabetes with consequences like heart disease, blindness, and possible amputations
- Atherosclerosis (hardening of the arteries) and the variety of associated cardiovascular conditions including heart attack and stroke
- Even osteoporosis and cancer

How is your risk tolerance now? Want more detail?

....

END NOTES

[1] Andrew Weil, "The Depression-Inflammation Connection," Huffington Post (November 4, 2011). Online at: http://www.huffingtonpost.com/andrew-weil-md/depression-and-inflammation_b_1071714.html (accessed February 20, 2014).

[2] "The Most Common Food Allergies: The Top 8," Eating With Food Allergies website (http://www.eatingwithfoodallergies.com/). Online at: http://www.eatingwithfoodallergies.com/commonfoodallergies.html (accessed February 25, 2014).

CHAPTER SEVEN

Sources of Inflammation

If I had known in my youth what I know now, I would be so much better off. As a teenager I idolized my father. Whatever he said, whatever he did, whatever he ate: I wanted to do the same thing too. I won't elaborate on how much trouble that caused me in school! I do want to tell you how I went astray on food, though.

We didn't eat much processed food in my house with the exception of bread (lots of white bread, the only kind available those days). But we made up for it by eating tons of white potatoes, the starchiest thing around. My idea of the perfect after-school snack was an iron skillet of American fried potatoes with onions and several slices of white bread slathered with butter. This was one of my father's favorite dishes as well—if you don't count fried chicken! In fact, potatoes were and, if I would allow it, would still be my all-time favorite food. Like everyone else, I thought of potatoes as just another vegetable.

While my mother and sister ate Brussels sprouts and cauliflower, my dad and I stuck to mashed potatoes and gravy with a generous side of white bread, also swimming in gravy. Green peas (which are actually pretty starchy, by the way) captured in a hollow amidst my mashed potatoes were as close to a real vegetable as I usually got.

Thanksgiving dinner was turkey, cornbread dressing, mashed potatoes, gravy, green bean casserole, white yeast rolls (oh, now I loved those rolls) and the requisite cranberry sauce out of a can. Dessert was lemon icebox pie, the only dessert my mother ever made. I prepared that very same meal for the next 40 years and really considered the green beans to be a "nod" to eating healthy. When my husband's grandmother (God rest her soul, she was a great cook) made us a pan of her famous yeast rolls, I sometimes ate every single one of them for my dinner and let other folks eat more reasonably.

The result of a meal heavy with carbs is an immediate need to take a nap. It's a symptom, I now know, of high blood sugar. Perhaps you've wondered why some folks nod off after Thanksgiving dinner? Well that's why! I shudder to think about the potential sugar levels attached to my (and my dad's) meals. Of course, neither of my parents nor anyone else's parents had a clue back in those days. We didn't understand the long-term consequences of the food choices we were making, and that's what I want to change for you right now. I want you to understand the health consequences of eating habits that lead to chronic inflammation in your body. If you didn't understand the connection between eating, diabetes, and cardiovascular disease before you picked up this book, I want you to be clear about it by the time you put this book down.

Omega-6 and Omega-3 Fatty Acids

Nutritional elements that we must eat in our food are called "essential." As we've seen, there are two essential polyunsaturated fatty acids derived by our bodies from fat that we eat. Omega-6 fatty acid, an essential fatty acid, is critical in support of the immune system. It provides for needed inflammation, blood clotting so you don't bleed to death, and cell production to heal damaged tissue. Good stuff when under control.

For balance, the body needs another essential fatty acid, omega-3, to reduce inflammation and lower fats in the bloodstream. In other words, omega-3 becomes important in restoring the body to working order after an infection. These two substances—omega-6 and omega-3—are partners in helping you to recover from illness, injury, or disease. After omega-6 has sounded the alarm and started your body's 911 response, omega-3 comes in and restores order once the emergency has been taken care of.

Let there be no mistake: both omega-6 and omega-3 are necessary. However, according to the University of Maryland Medical Center, the typical American diet tends to contain 14 to 25 times more omega-6 fatty acids than omega-3 fatty acids. The recommended diet ratio would be 4:1 or less.[1] That means we are much better equipped to create inflammation than we are to eliminate it! And that's a problem. On the one hand, we need inflammation in order for our immune system to work. On the other hand, we need for the inflammation to go away. The big question is, do we need to have less inflammation or should we just do a better job of getting rid of the inflammation we have?

The answer is YES. Both need to happen. Here is why: There is no shortage of omega-6 and it is difficult to imagine anyone having a deficiency of it. Omega-6 is found, in abundance, in almost every natural food source. That includes meat, starches, vegetables, and fruit. The big cause of an overabundance of dietary omega-6 is not due to the amount of it we get in natural foods. Instead, it is because of all the new and concentrated sources of omega-6 created by the industrial food revolution—sources like grain oils and processed foods.

Most grains have extraordinarily high levels of omega-6 and only a small amount of omega-3. (A cultivar of rapeseed known to us as canola would be an exception.) Properly prepared and eaten in reasonable proportions with other foods, grains are very nutritious and not usually an issue. But when grain and the oils extracted from grain became part of almost every processed food on the grocery and pantry shelf, the average American began consuming extraordinary levels of omega-6.

Conversely, while there is a little omega-3 in most foods, meat and coldwater fish are the usual significant sources. And the industrial food revolution has managed to reduce the available omega-3 in those sources by creating commercial cattle feedlots and fish farms which all use grains for feed. Grass-fed animals and wild caught fish are splendid sources of omega-3. Grain-fed animals like beef and farm-raised fish are not. See the problem?

There are only two significant but rarely consumed plant sources of omega-3: flax and chia seed. These are highly nutritious seeds, but you would have to eat quite a lot of them to meet your body's total requirement for omega-3.[2] The George Mateljan Foundation's "World's Healthiest Foods" website (www. whfood.org) describes the nutritional value of flax seed as well as flax seed oil.[3] I've used that website quite a bit; I really appreciate its depth and guidance on nutrition and food preparation.

As I mentioned before, omega-3 needs partners in the inflammation reduction game, partners like vitamins, antioxidants, anti-inflammatories, and other phytonutrients. Major sources are fruits and vegetables, and we don't eat nearly as many of these as we should. Here's the bottom line: We have to consume less omega-6 (lots less) and more omega-3 in (especially) fish along with vitamins and other nutrients in vegetables and fruit to achieve balance and help resolve chronic, ongoing inflammation.

Balancing omega-6 and omega-3 is not quite enough, though. We have to stop doing extra damage to ourselves as well.

Acid

If you are a gardener, you are probably familiar with measuring the acid or pH level in soil. Azaleas, as an example, require acidic soil to grow well. Unlike azaleas, the human body's desired condition is a pH balance between alkaline and acid, leaning slightly to the alkaline side. Maintaining the proper pH balance in the blood is your body's first priority and, if necessary, your system will use up your body's alkaline mineral stores in order to neutralize the acidity.

Where are those alkaline mineral stores? Why, in your bones and teeth, of course. When the acid level in your blood starts to go up, the body calls for calcium, a chief mineral reserve, and extracts it from your bones.

The acid in your body can come from a number of sources. These include:

- Chemical fertilizers and pesticides
- Artificial hormones we feed animals to make them produce more milk or grow larger
- Chemical additives and preservatives in processed food
- Chemically produced food substitutes
- Drugs (medically needed or recreational)

It's not as if we undergo a one-time exposure to such things. We keep absorbing these toxins every day, repeatedly, because they are so prevalent in the foods we consume. As acid builds up, the immune system will keep trying but ultimately fail to neutralize the acid. Then inflammation can become chronic. When that happens, chronic inflammation becomes the new "normal" in your life.

Take an organ transplant as an example. The assistant pastor of my church, a saint if ever there was one, was a double lung transplant recipient and lived many years in loving service. However, his immune system waged a mighty battle trying to reject the foreign lungs in his body. Highly acidic drugs were required to prevent total organ rejection. Inflammation throughout his body became chronic as a result of that medicine; he was in and out of the hospital regularly with conditions caused not by the lungs but by the drugs. When he died, it was not from lung failure. Instead, his kidneys and other bodily organs eventually gave out due to the trauma from all that inflammation caused by his medicine.

Equally important sources of acid are emotional stress (a big source) and the food we eat. As Dr. Theodore Baroody explains in his book Alkalize or Die, the foods we eat and other stressors fall into a range of acid or alkaline residue left in the body—not the taste of the food but the ash that is left as the food digests (or "burns").[4] As examples, lemons are acidic outside the body but they, in fact, form an alkaline ash when digested. Meat is alkaline on your plate but becomes very acidic when digested.

Emotional stress, meats, all processed foods (including refined white sugar and anything made of flour like breads, pastas, pastries, cakes, etc.) along with drugs, caffeinated drinks (coffee and cola), and cigarettes are on the extreme high end of the acid scale.

Love and kindness, as well as fruits and vegetables such as greens and berries, are the most alkaline things out there. Everything else such as whole grain, cheese, and dried beans is in the middle. Under proper eating circumstances you balance high acid content with alkaline content in your food. (Dr. Baroody recommends 20% acid to 80% alkaline, but that is a condition probably achievable only by raw vegans.)

Examine the points above carefully. Most of the food the average American eats, especially including the food products created by the processed food industry, are all on the high acidity list. All the alkaline fruits and vegetables that would neutralize acid are the foods least eaten by Americans. It is pretty easy to see how we might be out of acid balance.

Look at this another way. As the history of the American diet over the last 100 years evolved, we collectively moved…

- from a historical and very practical diet with minimal high acid-producing foods like meat, a good amount of neutral acidity foods like beans, and lots of alkaline-producing foods like fresh vegetables,

- to today's commercially profitable diet containing significant amounts of high acid-producing foods like meat, along with a bunch of processed refined grains and sugar, with tons of chemically created stuff like artificial sweeteners, tobacco, alcohol, and recreational and medicinal drugs to top it all off. And, of course, we've gradually decreased our intake of alkaline-producing foods along the way.

Now we have the combined effect of too much acid added to an imbalance of omega-6 / omega-3 fatty acids. It's not a good combination. And it's not all we're dealing with now, either.

Trans-Fats

This brings us to those nasty, process-created trans-fats. The label on a processed food package frequently lists "partially hydrogenated (insert name) oil." You saw earlier that hydrogenation is a heat and chemical process that converts polyunsaturated fats (usually grain oils) to a higher degree of saturation for use in commercial processed foods. Unfortunately, hydrogenation creates trans-fats that are very dangerous to the body.

Products using partially hydrogenated oils became more common during World War II when butter was rationed and margarine appeared on the scene. Then the government and some outfits like the American Heart Association, with the enthusiastic support of the vegetable oil manufacturers, campaigned for cutting back on cholesterol and saturated fats in the belief that these were the causes of rampant cardiovascular disease. Partially hydrogenated vegetable oil began appearing in just about all processed foods. Eventually, under pressure, fast food restaurants stopped using saturated fats like lard and palm oil for frying and began using partially hydrogenated oils. Then in the 1990s the bad news about hydrogenation came to light.[5]

Now, 100 years after the introduction of Crisco shortening, the processed food and fast food industries scramble to eliminate hydrogenated or partially hydrogenated oils, better known now as trans-fats. This is why New York City banned trans-fats in restaurants in 2006, an event that got a lot of press at the time.

Trans-fats are deadly. They disturb your body's cell structure in ugly ways.[6]According to the Mayo Clinic, trans-fats also increase triglycerides (free fat in your blood) and lead to inflammation, thus promoting plaque buildup in the arteries.[7]Do you see how the list of the sources of inflammation keeps getting longer? We now have the combined effect of an imbalance of omega-6/omega-3 fatty acids, too much acid, and those nasty trans-fats all piled on top of one another. But that's still not all.

Blood Sugar and Insulin

The human body's primary energy source is glucose, known to most of us as sugar. Glucose is usually made available in our blood from carbohydrates we eat, and the amount of glucose in the blood is also related to inflamed blood vessel walls. In addition to extracting glucose from carbohydrates, we can also draw our energy from stored body fat. We'll look at body fat in the section on Excess Body Fat below. Here, let's take a look at carbs. Carbohydrates include:

- Starchy carbohydrates like beans, grains, and root vegetables such as potatoes

- Vegetables and fruit

Generally, all carbohydrates digest into a combination of fructose and glucose. Fructose will become important when we talk about body fat. We want to focus on glucose at this point.

The body keeps a maintenance-level amount of glucose in the blood at all times. When the blood's glucose rises above maintenance-level (like when you eat a meal), the hormone insulin is released by the pancreas in order to escort the glucose from the blood stream to our body cells (muscles, fat, and liver). Some portion of that glucose will be stored in a rainy day supply called glycogen in the liver, muscles, and, to a small degree, other organs. The glucose not immediately used for energy or to restore the glycogen supply goes to fat—literally.

Conversely, when the glucose level in the blood falls too low (like between meals, or when sleeping or exercising), another hormone causes the glycogen stored in the liver to be released into the blood stream to restore normal glucose levels. That same hormone also triggers the release of fatty acids from your fat cells, making energy available for the body.

So in the simplest possible terms, in the absence of insulin in the bloodstream, the body depends on glycogen stores and body fat for energy. When the blood stream is rife with glucose and insulin, the body will use glucose almost exclusively for fuel, storing most of the excess as fat. In any case, remember that insulin is required in order to move glucose into the cells for energy.

What matters with insulin and glucose, as it relates to inflammation (and sometimes type 2 diabetes) are three main factors:

- How quickly the carbohydrates you eat are converted to glucose
- How high your blood sugar goes in that process (the spike)
- How long your blood sugar remains elevated

Vegetables and fruit, sometimes known as simple carbohydrates, include a lot of water as well as fiber and the amount of sugar in each serving is small. The glucose conversion is quick but the risk of a spike is minimal.

Even simple carbs are not created equal, though. The advantages of minimal sugar and lots of fiber present in vegetables and (especially) fruit are lost in juices. Squeeze the juice out of several oranges and throw the rest away and what is left in the glass is a pile of tasty sugar—thus the digestion is quick and the blood sugar impact can be significant. Plain refined table sugar (sucrose) is also a simple carb but, as with juices, has nothing to slow digestion of the glucose and contains no nutrition whatsoever. Any food containing a significant amount of table sugar, often pastries of some sort, can cause a spike in blood sugar very quickly.

Then there are the starches, vegetables where the amount and structure of the sugar is more complex. Pinto beans, as an example of a complex carb, have lots of sugar in the form of starch but also include high levels of protein and fiber. The starch is complex and takes a bit longer to breakdown into simple sugar. Protein digests slowly and, along with fiber, interferes with and spreads the sugar digestion out over time, helping to avoid spikes. Grain and root vegetables also have a lot of starch but the sugar structure is somewhat less complex and digests more quickly. Also, the amount of protein and fiber is lower than in beans.

Note also that the bulk of the fiber in a potato is in the skin. Excess potatoes, usually eaten without the skin, are the downfall of many a diet. Here is a comparison to help you understand: A serving of baked potato with the skin (one small red potato which most of us would consider a ridiculously small amount) contains 29 grams of carb with only 6 grams of protein and fiber.[8] A serving of kidney beans (about ½ cup) has 23 grams of carb with 15 grams of protein and fiber.[9] So obviously, beans are going to digest more slowly and be less prone to spike blood sugar. You can get this kind of data for just about any food available on the market today at the Nutrition Data website, which is a personal favorite of mine (www.nutritiondata.self.com).

When extra protein, fat, and fiber are consumed in combination with carbohydrate foods, like if you add a ham hock with the beans and include a salad, sugar digestion can be slowed even more. The better the meal balance, the less chance of a blood sugar spike.

In whole form, all carbohydrates are healthy and nutritious. The big trouble starts when we consume them in refined, processed form—to make it simple that means things like chips, French fries, and all foods made from flour and refined sugar. These are the foods that drive high and potentially continuous levels of blood sugar.

Consider the typical tortilla chip, which is made from refined grain. Once it is ground up, the complex sugar structure in wheat grain is broken down. Most of the nutrition and fiber are gone; the carbohydrates fast forward through normal digestion and become, effectively, simple sugar. And lots of it. When we make a cake, adding refined sugar (that used to be a nutritious beet, by the way) to the flour (grain that has been ground into sugar), we end up with a serious pile of sugar. Large amounts of simple sugar digest immediately and hightail it for your blood stream, screaming for insulin along the way.

The occasional blood sugar spike is not the problem. There is likely to be a spike after you eat that big piece of chocolate birthday cake. The problem is that some of us eat these foods every day, at every meal, in between meals, and in excess. Half sack of crackers, chips, or cookies; a slice (or two) of cake, a nice big bowl of macaroni and cheese, or (my personal favorite) a double order of fries. Thus, the amount of "energy" or sugar arriving in the blood stream for handling comes in such large doses and happens so often that blood sugar can spike and remain high. When this happens, three major problems can occur:

- The body cells just plain get full, no more room in the inn, and resist the glucose. The liver sees that that blood sugar is just hanging around in the blood stream and instructs the pancreas to ship out more and more insulin, trying to force the body cells to accept the glucose. The pancreas, weakened by this extra demand, becomes less and less able to produce insulin. Some combination of these two conditions (and sometimes others) will be diagnosed as diabetes.

- The excess sugar in the blood coats protein in the blood vessels walls creating things called AGEs: advanced glycation end products. AGEs release free radicals which damage everything they touch, including the blood vessels themselves. The damage to even small veins and capillaries helps explain why diabetics are susceptible to blindness and amputations. Damage to arteries, on the other hand, plays into cardiovascular disease. One helpful thing is that sugar also accumulates on red blood cells so it is possible to determine how high, on average, your blood sugar has been with a simple blood test called A1c. A red blood cell lives three or so months before dying and being replaced by a new one so there is always a fresh opportunity to see how you are doing, blood sugar wise. Measurement of A1c is important in diagnosing and treating diabetes.

- The excess sugar can also join together with LDL cholesterol particles in the blood, also creating AGEs. While LDL cholesterol, usually known as "bad cholesterol," has an important role in delivery of cholesterol to the body's cells, it is also very susceptible to oxidation. A recent study from the American Diabetes Association describes the process this way: "AGEs can modify LDL cholesterol in such a way that it tends to become easily oxidized and deposited within vessel walls, causing streak formation and, in time, atheroma."[10] Two things can happen with glycated LDL: First, the glycated LDL releases those rotten free radicals, further damaging the blood vessel; secondly, the LDL cholesterol stops doing its main job which is feeding cholesterol to the body cells.[11] So instead, the damaged LDL just floats around making itself available to be absorbed into the damaged blood vessel (into the very damage it helped create in the first place!), which is part of the stuff that plaque is made of.

- Along with other things, your HDL cholesterol (sometimes called "good cholesterol") is supposed to sweep up all this trash and carry it away. But perhaps you have an overload of damaged LDL and, by chance, your HDL cholesterol is also low. That's not uncommon, actually. If that happens, then you've got problems. So the logic behind reducing your LDL cholesterol is that the fewer LDL particles you have, the fewer there are to be damaged and get stuck, thus minimizing the accumulation of plaque in blood vessels. It is the plaque that is characteristic of atherosclerosis.

Atherosclerosis is a condition that affects medium and larger arteries. It occurs when fat, cholesterol, and other substances build up in the walls of arteries and form hard structures called plaque. This build up occurs when the arteries are damaged—which can be one result of persistently high blood sugar—and the immune system does what it does best: causes blood clots to stop bleeding, generates inflammation in the healing process, and creates plaque to seal over the damage. Get the picture? Put high blood sugar, inflammation, damaged blood vessels and LDL cholesterol together and you'll eventually get atherosclerosis. (See Atherosclerosis later on in this book for more information.) It is not a condition you want to have.

If, by chance, you've skipped past the last few paragraphs because they just sounded too complicated, or words like advanced glycation end products and free radicals caused brain freeze, then I hope you will stop here and re-read them. I could have just said, "Keep your blood sugar down if you can 'cause it's good for you." That would have used a lot fewer words. And you could have just said, "Well, I'll try but, you know, I love my bread and I just have to eat lots of it," with no understanding of the possible cost. Like I said at the beginning of this chapter, I really want you to understand the consequences of certain eating habits on your long-term health. I want you to get a good grasp on the connection between eating, diabetes, and cardiovascular disease. Believe me: it's worth the trouble of finding out.

Excess Body Fat

Let's start with the part that isn't fair. We each arrived on this earth with a different set of genes. Some of those genes define how much fat we tend to accumulate and where. Some of the people you know are naturally lean and full of energy and they will be that way almost regardless of what or how much they eat. They just burn those calories off. More often than not, they have at least one parent with the same characteristics. Others, however, aren't so genetically lucky. They gain weight just by looking at a donut or piece of chocolate cake. Their metabolism is just naturally slower. They put on pounds easily and struggle ever to shed them.

That doesn't mean that the lean folks who eat poorly won't be impacted by their diet. It just means that impact may not show up in body fat. As a person who is both diabetic and naturally lean, I am a perfect example.

So the lean among us are usually more energetic and more active and literally burn more calories from both food and body fat every day. These are the people who never sit down, the people who jog five miles every day just because they want to. Unfortunately, none of us gets to choose our own metabolism. But slim or rotund, all of us have some level of body fat worth learning about.

Although our body requires the nutrition in fat for many valuable purposes, a primary job of dietary fat (the fat in food) is to generate back-up energy for us in the form of body fat. But when it comes to excess body fat, it usually isn't the fat in the diet that creates the excess. According to many experts on fat and its impact on our health, we don't accumulate that fat around our middles just by chowing down on fat in our food.[12] We get fat by eating excessive amounts of refined starchy carbohydrates and sugar just like those gorillas in the London Zoo did.

As I mentioned before, over two-thirds of Americans are either overweight or obese. Have you ever noticed how we are bombarded with messages about the importance of reducing fat in order to lose weight at every turn? We're told the key is in eating low fat cheese, milk, and meats, along with low fat processed food you find on the shelf at the grocery. Celebrity chefs on talk shows and famous doctors can be seen at every click on the remote touting the value of reduced fat. Just recently I watched a TV chef making "Oreo truffles" out of crushed Oreo cookies, low-fat cream cheese, and almond bark. He made a big deal of the low fat cream cheese and skipped over the real issue: the overwhelming amount of sugar in Oreos and almond bark!

Excess body fat, especially around the middle, causes inflammation issues to double up. The extra body fat around your butt or thighs, as an example, may not look particularly good but the fat around your middle is a different kind of fat called visceral, the really dangerous stuff. The presence of too much visceral fat is common in a condition referred to as metabolic syndrome, a combination of conditions that you don't want.

If you think about it, this idea of carbohydrate sugar as the source of body fat will make sense. You have heard, no doubt, of the Atkins Diet.[13] A meat and fat diet and a weight loss plan, this diet starts out eliminating all carbohydrates except a handful of leafy green vegetables a day and then adds vegetables and fruits back over time until you stop losing weight. Whether your doctor approves of this diet or not, people do lose weight despite the significant amount of fat in the diet.

Of course, people also lose weight on the McDougall Plan, a low-fat vegan diet with no meat at all.[14] And people lose weight on the Ornish diet as well, a low-fat vegetarian diet.[15] Now, however can this be? How can both the Atkins Diet (a plan for big-time carnivores, which includes lots of fat) and the McDougall and Ornish diets (plans aimed at big-time vegetarians or vegans, which minimize fat) both lead to weight loss? The reason is because one characteristic common to all three diets is the discouragement of processed refined foods made from white flour and sugar.[16] Reduce those carbs, and you reduce the glucose levels in the blood and the accumulation of body fat.

Also of importance in weight gain but in a different way is the amount of fructose in our diets. This raises the question of the day: Is high fructose corn syrup, HFCS, bad for us or not? The answer is yes, but, in truth, if it weren't for the fact that it is chemically and heat processed, it wouldn't be much worse for you than plain old sugar.

Refined white table sugar (sucrose) is about half fructose and half glucose. Fructose in some partnership with glucose naturally occurs in all fruit, and is present, usually in small amounts, in vegetables. Both fructose and glucose have a sweet taste but the more fructose, the sweeter. In fact, it seems that extra sweetness is addictive, making the consumer crave still more.

Once eaten, however, fructose and glucose take different paths in the body. Glucose becomes blood sugar and an immediate source of energy. Fructose, on the other hand, has to be metabolized by the liver and does not directly impact blood sugar. What the liver does with the fructose depends on the condition of the liver's glycogen store, the rainy day supply of glucose mentioned in the section on Blood Sugar. If the liver's glycogen store is full, the fructose is converted into triglyceride fat by the liver and shipped to the body's fat cells. If the glycogen store is not full, the liver will first use some fructose to fill up the glycogen store before sending any balance to fat storage.

Consider for a minute your own personal glycogen store. Is it likely to be empty? Not if you are eating an excess of carbohydrates (which most of us are). So you can probably plan on your fructose making its way to fat cell storage.

High fructose corn syrup (HFCS), a common commercially produced sweetener created from corn, was initially believed to be a good thing for diabetics because fructose does not impact blood sugar. But just like refined sugar, HFCS also contains both glucose and fructose—although it sometimes contains a higher percentage of fructose than other sugars. Because fructose is sweeter, then, less is required and HFCS is cheaper than refined sugar. That explains why it commonly appears in processed foods including soft drinks. Consuming soft drinks, as you know, is a favorite American pastime. Addictive, perhaps?

The words "commonly appears" are at the heart of the problem with HFCS and, in fact, all sugar. In the old, old days, say in the early 1900's, before much commercially processed food, we ate the sugar in fruit and we used refined white sugar for special occasions when it was available. Any food processing, be that cooking, canning, or grinding, occurred in your great, great, grandmother's kitchen. Otherwise we ate the food as God delivered it in the plant growing out of the ground. The liver had no trouble back then handling the required fructose-to-fat conversion because the amount of fructose in a diet was low. Consequently the impact on body fat was minimal and few people were overweight.

Above my china cabinet hangs a picture labeled "Arkansas on Wheels Trip to Mount Vernon" dated 1916. There are 51 men and women in this picture, adults in their 40's and 50s, among them my husband's grandfather. Beyond two men I would described as husky, there are no overweight people.

Just recently I saw a 1939 video of the streets of New York.[17] The streets are packed with people of every age, sex, and race and the absence of excess body fat in the people is striking.

Moving forward to 1959, I carefully studied the yearbook for my junior year in high school. Out of my class of 258, there were two girls who were slightly heavy along with one teacher. The other three classes fit the same model; there were essentially no overweight people in my entire school.

Skip ahead to today. Wander over to Wal-Mart or your local high school tomorrow and take a look. We don't need a report to tell us that excess weight among adults, teens, and even children is common.

The commercial food industry has changed things dramatically. These days there is sugar and/or HFCS in almost everything on the grocery shelf, either added to improve the taste since processing has a tendency to remove the taste or as a substitute for the fat removed in the interest of making the food "low fat." Add to that the extraordinary amounts of soft drinks Americans consume—which are also "low fat" but absolutely loaded with sugar.

The current overload of fructose in the American diet can overwhelm the liver, interfering with other liver functions and causing excess fat production. In his book, The McDougall Program, Dr. John McDougall writes of a patient who had to cut fruit out of his diet because his triglycerides (fat in the blood) were too high—even though there is no fat in fruit.[18]

I hope the picture I'm painting is clear. If you are a heavy consumer of sugar, regardless of what form of sugar, you are a heavy consumer of fructose. This is true when you are baking a cake in your own kitchen, putting a processed salad dressing on your salad, or chugging a soft drink. Not only is that excess fructose placing a heavy burden on your liver, arguably the most important organ in your body outside of your heart, but also likely to make its way directly to your fat cells. It is not by happenstance that two-thirds of Americans are overweight and it seems to have little to do with the amount of fat that they eat.

Finally, beyond the causes of excess body fat, the very existence of that fat hanging around your belly creates even more inflammation according to the American Heart Association as well as researchers at the Walter and Liza Hall Institute in Melbourne, Australia. Researcher Professor Len Harrison writes, "The complications of obesity such as insulin resistance and diabetes, cardiovascular disease associated with hardening of the arteries, and liver problems are the result of inflammation that occurs in the (visceral) fat tissue."[19]

And so we have almost reached the end. To an imbalance of omega-6/omega-3 fatty acids, excess body acid, trans-fats, and excess blood sugar we have now added excess body fat as the final of the five major dietary contributors to inflammation and chronic, deadly diseases in Americans. But there is one more important contributor for about 19% of us—smoking.

Smoking

The 19% of Americans who smoke are in a special pickle.[20] When I was a kid we were told that smoking caused lung cancer. And since I knew of people with lung cancer who never smoked, the risk seemed to me to be exaggerated. Now I know that inflammation from smoking is a far more serious risk. According to the American Journal of Physiology, cigarette smoking causes inflammation in the arteries and, perhaps surprisingly, "the cardiovascular morbidity and mortality induced by cigarette smoking exceed those attributable to lung cancer."[21]

Smoking is another, equally dangerous contributor to any and all conditions marked by inflamed arteries. But it isn't just the smoking; it is the smoking along with stress and food acids, trans-fats, high blood sugar, excess body fat, as well as too much omega-6 and not enough omega-3 in our diet. In simpler terms, if you have the consequences of a really bad diet and you smoke too, Lord help you.

....

END NOTES

[1] "Omega-6 fatty acids," from the Complementary and Alternative Medicine Guide [online] of the University of Maryland Medical Center. Online at: http://www.umm.edu/altmed/articles/omega-6-000317.htm (accessed February 25, 2014).

[2] See the later chapter on "Cholesterol and Saturated Fat" for a more complete explanation on this issue.

[3] George Mateljan Foundation, "What's New and Beneficial About Flaxseeds." Online at: http://whfoods.org/genpage.php?tname=foodspice&dbid=81 (accessed February 25, 2014); and "Chia or flax seeds: Which is preferable as an addition to my meals?" Online at: http://www.whfoods.com/genpage.php?tname=dailytip&dbid=242 (accessed February 25, 2014).

[4] Theodore Baroody, Alkalize or Die (Holographic Health Press, 1991).

[5] American Heart Association, "A History of Trans Fat," AHA Website [www.heart.org] (August, 2010). Online at: http://www.heart.org/HEARTORG/GettingHealthy/FatsAndOils/Fats101/A-History-of-Trans-Fat_UCM_301463_Article.jsp#.TydmMYEU7To (accessed February 25, 2014).

[6] Sally Fallon with Mary G. Enig, Nourishing Traditions: The Cookbook that Challenges Politically Correct Nutrition and the Diet Dictocrats (Washington, DC: New Trends Publishing, Inc., 2001).

[7] Mayo Clinic Staff, "Trans fat is double trouble for your heart health," Mayo Clinic (August 6, 2014). Online at: http://www.mayoclinic.com/health/trans-fat/CL00032 (accessed October 3, 2014).

[8] Information from the Nutrition Data website: "Potato, baked, flesh and skin, without salt," Online at: http://nutritiondata.self.com/facts/vegetables-and-vegetable-products/2770/2 (accessed February 25, 2014).

9   Information from the Nutrition Data website: "Beans, kidney, all types, mature seeds, cooked, boiled, without salt," online at: http://nutritiondata. self.com/facts/legumes-and-legume-products/4297/2 (accessed February 25, 2014).

10   Melpomeni Peppa, Jaime Uribarri, and Helen Vlassara, "Glucose, Advanced Glycation End Products, and Diabetes Complications: What Is New and What Works," Clinical Diabetes 21:4 (2003): 186-187. Online at: http://clinical.diabetesjournals.org/content/21/4/186.full (accessed February 25, 2014).

11   According to Life Extension, "[O]nce LDL has become glycated it is no longer recognized by the LDL receptor on cell surfaces, meaning that it will remain in circulation and is more likely to contribute to the atherosclerotic process" ("Cholesterol Management," Life Extension: Foundation for Longer Life (©1995-2014). Online at: https://www.lef.org/ protocols/heart_circulatory/cholesterol_management_01.htm (accessed February 25, 2014).

12   The YouTube video is available via KimKomando's website: http://videos. komando.com/watch/3386/viral-videos-incredible-color-footage-of-1939-new-york (accessed February 25, 2014).

13   McDougall, The McDougall Program.

14   See the Walter and Eliza Hall Institute, "Obesity and diabetes: Immune cells in fat tissue explain the link," ScienceDaily (November 8, 2010). Online at: www.sciencedaily.com/releases/2010/08/100816095800.htm (accessed February 25, 2014).

15   Centers for Disease Control and Prevention, "Smoking and Tobacco Use". Online at: http://www.cdc.gov/tobacco/data_statistics/fact_sheets/ fast_facts/ (accessed February 25, 2014).

16   Zsuzsanna Orosz, et al., "Cigarette smoke-induced proinflammatory alterations in the endothelial phenotype: role of NAD(P)H oxidase activation," American Journal of Physiology 292:1 (January 2007): H130-H139. Online at: http://ajpheart.physiology.org/content/292/1/ H130.full (accessed February 25, 2014).

CHAPTER EIGHT

Calories

I am betting you have already figured out that counting calories may not be required. For one thing, it is darn hard to do. Get yourself a fancy app for your iPhone and be meticulous about entering everything you eat. Buy yourself a book that includes the calories in all the food you can think of and don't eat a bite until you look it up. Not me! That is part of the reason that diets equipped with prepackaged food seem to work so well; somebody else decided what food to include and determined the serving sizes. (At least those diets work until you stop buying the prepackaged food and find yourself out there all on your own.)

To be blunt, the idea of counting calories at every meal for the rest of your life is just, well, not very pleasant.

The information in this book makes it pretty clear that all calories are not created equal. Jonny Bowden, Ph.D., a board-certified nutritionist and author, explains this fact: "Study after study shows that diets based on the same amount of calories, but different proportions of fat, protein and carbohydrates, result in different amounts of weight loss."[1] Or weight gain, of course.

Research conducted over many years at the Harvard School of Public Health reinforces Dr. Bowden's view with more detail. Those findings showed the foods that caused the greatest weight gain were potatoes in all forms, sugary drinks and sweet desserts, red meat, refined grains, and other fried foods. Not a big surprise, except I haven't yet figured out how red meat fits in. (I suspect it may be connected to the food usually eaten with red meat but the study data is not in sufficient detail to show that.) The stuff that resulted in weight loss was fruits, vegetables, and whole grains. Just as we should expect. But the big bang difference was that "an increased intake of dairy products, whether low-fat (milk) or full-fat (milk and cheese), had a neutral effect on weight. And despite conventional advice to eat less fat, weight loss was greatest among people who ate more yogurt and nuts, including peanut butter, over each four-year period."[2] In other words, generally speaking those starches and processed foods that generate the greatest blood sugar will cause weight gain. Those natural foods that are neutral, like vegetables and such, and those that slow down blood sugar, like some protein and fat, are likely to cause weight loss (or prevent weight gain.)

On this basis, the only other directions you need to consider, beyond those already detailed in my chapter on The Almost Perfect Diet and explained in detail in the sections that followed, have to do with the recommended number and size of servings per day in each food category. In case you're wondering, here they are:

- Six to eight one-ounce equivalent servings of protein including a mix of meat, full fat milk, yogurt, cheese, beans, and nuts. For this purpose, we are not including vegetables although they are usually protein sources to a small degree. An equivalent is:

  - 1 ounce of meat 1 egg
  - ½ cup of milk or yogurt (unsweetened)
  - 2 ounces of cheese
  - 1 ounce of nuts
  - ½ cup of beans

- A maximum of two servings of starch (whole grain and potatoes) in any form per meal, six total per day. An equivalent is:

  - 1 thin slice of bread
  - ¼ - ½ cup dry cereal
  - ½ cup cooked cereal
  - 1 small pancake
  - 1 new potato

- All the vegetables you can eat along with 2 to 3 pieces of fruit.

- The amount of oil that is needed for taste, sauté, or dressing, not for frying.

If you are going to err, then err on the side of more vegetables. The rules in my game will otherwise have to do with eating the right fats, protein, and grains. This is going to be way easier than counting calories.

A disclaimer right now for those lucky people who don't gain weight. While the other rules are the same, the number of servings can change with minimal impact. These folks just have a different metabolism (lucky for them!). As for children, remember that they are growing. As a consequence, their caloric needs can be significantly more than their size would suggest. Given the proper food, they will usually eat only as much as they need. But filled up with refined grains and processed foods, a child can be perpetually hungry, undernourished, and eventually overweight.

....

END NOTES

[1] Quoted in Jenny Stamos Kovacs, "The Dos and Don'ts of Counting Calories," WebMD feature (2007). Online at: http://www.webmd.com/diet/features/dos-donts-counting-calories (accessed December 17, 2014).

[2] Jane E. Brody, "Still Counting Calories? Your Weight-Loss Plan May Be Outdated," New York Times (July 18, 2011). Online at: http://www.nytimes.com/2011/07/19/health/19brody.html?pagewanted=all&_r=0 (accessed December 17, 2014).

CHAPTER NINE

Which Diet Will You Choose?

So here we are. We all need to choose a healthy diet. And we don't need a diet to gain or lose a few pounds but rather a diet to live with throughout our lives. So assuming you are not anxious to be diabetic or looking forward to your first (or second) heart attack, the following offers the high points of various dietary alternatives. As you read remember this, think carefully before choosing any diet that absolutely requires taking supplements regardless of your age and health condition. I simply don't believe a healthy and holistic diet should require pill-based supplements at all — if we're talking about an otherwise healthy individual.

You may choose to be a herbivore that eats plants only, a carnivore that eats meat only, or an omnivore that eats both. There are, by the way, variations of each of these.

A human herbivore is usually called a vegan. Vegans don't eat any animal products whatsoever. They consume only plant foods. This diet is a bit harder to follow than it sounds. For example, even jello would not be on a vegan's menu because gelatin is actually an animal product. Vegans get their protein from starches like legumes (beans) and grains as well as a small portion from the vegetables in their diets.

Some vegans avoid animal food out of concern for the truly horrible treatment of animals in commercial feedlots. Others don't want to eat meat that has been contaminated in feedlots. Still others care more about the pollution and consumption of natural resources like topsoil and water that is associated with raising meat. The Food Revolution by John Robbins and the Omnivore's Dilemma by Michael Pollan are two of several books providing detailed analysis of these conditions.

Some vegans, however, believe strongly that a plant-based, low fat diet is the healthiest. Several doctors like John McDougall of The McDougall Program and Dean Ornish of the Preventive Medicine Research Institute, have entirely or almost entirely vegan, low-fat programs known for reversing serious illness. Once the arteries are well clogged, extraordinary measures may be required.

Other vegans, however, think that a diet full of processed, high carbohydrate foods and sugar meets the standard simply because it doesn't include meat. Not long ago I joined a group at a lunch buffet. Among the group was an overweight woman I knew to be an espoused vegan. She ate potato salad, tater tots, fried okra, rolls, and a bit of salad. She rounded that off with a piece of cherry pie. It is certainly possible to be overweight and undernourished at the same time on a vegan diet.

Those considering a vegan diet should remember this: Of the dietary essential nutrients required by the human body, two are totally absent or inadequate from a vegan diet – vitamin B12 and to some degree omega-3 fatty acids. Special supplements developed from non-animal sources are required to make up for B12 deficiency. Omega-3 is a little more complicated. It actually comes in three subcategory forms.[1] They include:

- ALA from plant foods like flax and to a lesser degree walnuts and green leafy vegetables.

- EPA, and DHA from meat (especially fish) and meat products like dairy and eggs.

EPA and DHA are sometimes listed as "essential," sometimes not. This is explained by WebMD. "Because essential fatty acids (ALA, DHA, EPA) are not made in the body or are inefficiently converted from ALA to EPA and DHA, we need to get them from our diet." For clarity, the body can convert ALA into EPA AND DHA but it takes a whole bunch of ALA to do the job.[2] This conversion limitation is magnified in a diet with insufficient ALA. Supplements made from seaweed (food sources of fish) are recommended for vegans.

From a weight perspective vegans also need to understand how important fat is on a vegan diet. If the blood stream is always full of sugar from refined grain and sugar consumption, no body fat is likely to be burned. A balanced vegan diet will include good natural sources of fat in the food and won't include refined grains, excessive starches like potatoes, and sugar.

Then there are vegetarians, folks who don't eat meat or eat only fish but do eat dairy and meat products like eggs, butter, milk, etc. As with vegans, vegetarians have a variety of reasons for preferring this diet. A vegetarian diet can be as deficient as any other if it is full of refined grains and sugar. But vegetarians do have an easier time getting fat and protein in their diets because of their willingness to eat eggs, milk, cheese, and other dairy products.[3]

Carnivores eat only meat and tend to be wild animals. Their diets do not contain any plant foods at all. I don't personally know any human carnivores. It is frankly hard to imagine a human being these days eating only meat and meat products!

The average American is an omnivore eating a diet that includes at least some meat and/or fish, fats, starches, vegetables, and fruit. The amount of each varies enormously by preference, culture, and habit. This diet provides a natural opportunity to consume all essential nutrients without benefit of supplements and provides the greatest variety of food choices—a natural opportunity often missed.

There are also a number of "programs" in the omnivore category. Dr. Atkins' New Diet Revolution, a meat-and-fat-heavy diet I mentioned in my section on "Blood Sugar and Insulin" (see the chapter, Sources of Inflammation) is one example.[4] The Atkins diet followed religiously is, by all reports, very effective at achieving weight loss. However the weight loss value is in the absence of carbohydrate, not the consumption of the meat/fat. If you aren't consuming any carbohydrates, there really isn't anything left to eat except meat and fat. The excessive amounts of acid in meat protein over a long-term basis have detrimental potential.

You might also consider The Anti-Inflammatory Diet by Dr. Andrew Weil,[5] and Eat Fat, Lose Fat by Dr. Mary Enig and Sally Fallon,[6] which I mentioned briefly in my section on "Excess Body Fat" (also in the chapter on Sources of

Inflammation). Typically all these diets place a particular positive emphasis on something — something like rice, meat, or fat. But what is most striking, at least to me, about these diets and others is that they almost invariably call for minimization or elimination of refined, processed grains and refined sugars.

Finally, there is the "Paleo diet" which, if followed religiously, essentially excludes all complex carbohydrates including grain and beans along with refined sugar. Another program, The Type-2 Diabetes Breakthrough by Dr. Frank Shallenberger, calls for close management of all starchy carbohydrates and sugar, refined or not, as sources of dietary glucose problematic to diabetics.[7] Note that Dr. McDougall, as a vegan and starch advocate, would argue with this type of management. But even his diet minimizes refined, processed grains and sugars.

Surely all of these experts can't be wrong about something in which they are all in agreement — that we must minimize or eliminate refined, processed grains and sugars. So let's assume, just for the sake of conversation, that you have become convinced through reading this book that some changes in your diet and lifestyle are in order but you are still worried by cholesterol and saturated fat. Fair enough. Let's take a look at these in greater depth.

....

END NOTES

1   "The Facts on Omega-3 Fatty Acids," WebMD fact sheet article (2013). (Reviewed by Melinda Ratini, DO, MS.) Online at: http://www.webmd. com/healthy-aging/omega-3-fatty-acids-fact-sheet (accessed February 25, 2014).

2   Joel Fuhrman, "What Vegans May be Missing," Dr. Fuhrman: Smart Nutrition, Superior Health website. Online at: http://www.drfuhrman. com/library/what_vegans_may_be_missing-DHA.aspx (accessed December 17, 2014).

3   As you might have guessed, the vegan woman described above is actually a vegetarian, although she probably doesn't know it. Her diet clearly contains animal products such as milk and eggs.

4   Robert C. Atkins, Dr. Atkins' New Diet Revolution (New York: HarperCollins, 2002).

5   Andrew Weil, "The Depression-Inflammation Connection," Huffington Post (November 4, 2011). Online at: http://www.huffingtonpost.com/andrew-weil-md/depression-and-inflammation_b_1071714.html (accessed February 20, 2014).

6   Mary Enig and Sally Fallon, Eat Fat, Lose Fat, Reprint edition (Plume, 2006).

7   Frank Shallenberger, The Type-2 Diabetes Breakthrough: A Revolutionary Approach to Treating Type-2 Diabetes (Laguna Beach, CA, Basic Health Publications, 2005).

CHAPTER TEN

Cholesterol and Saturated Fat

Despite the press given to the need to reduce consumption of cholesterol and saturated fat in meats, we all need to understand that the body requires, I repeat, requires both. The body, primarily the liver, can actually make all we need— which is the reason that a vegan diet is even possible. (If you haven't figured it out yet, without your liver you are in deep trouble!) When all is working properly, the liver adjusts its cholesterol and fat production based on your diet. Any excess cholesterol hanging around is swept out in body waste.

So on the surface it looks like we might not need to eat any cholesterol or saturated fat at all, right? I mean, if the liver will make all you need, why eat it? There are reasons.

Your liver cannot make vitamin B12 or omega-3 fatty acids, both essential, which means we have to consume them in food. Usable vitamin B12 is found only in meat, which includes fish, the most significant source of omega-3. We can't eat meat without also getting cholesterol and saturated fat, and we can become B12 and even omega-3 deficient if we don't eat meat. So it takes some meat (although a lot less than you probably think) to meet your need for vitamin B12 and probably omega-3. It is really that simple.

Why would it be arranged this way?

For much of the world's population (both today and in the distant past) meat is hard to obtain and is not daily fare. Meat, of course, is chock full of protein. Since a daily supply of protein is required for your body, the good Lord provided an alternate source in plants. That makes getting plenty of protein possible even without meat. It's similar with our body's Vitamin A needs. A daily supply of vitamin A is both essential and found in meat, but there's a backup plan in the compound beta carotene. Found only in plants, beta carotene is easily converted to vitamin A by the body when required.[1]

It's a little different when it comes to vitamin B12. Instead of providing an alternate source of B12, the good Lord arranged for a stored supply in the body. And it's a supply that gets replenished when meat is available. If we eliminate meat completely from our diet, we can eventually use up our stored supply of B12. Of course, we live a lot longer now than we once did. B12 deficiency in older people is quite common, sometimes because they don't metabolize their nutrients very well.

Like protein and vitamin A, the body also needs an ongoing, not occasional, supply of cholesterol and saturated fat. This helps us to understand why the liver can either make all the cholesterol and saturated fat we need or adjust its production when we have both in our diet. Cholesterol and saturated fat are in meat, the meat that might be in short supply.

One issue not too different from a deficiency of meat in the diet is the inability to digest meat efficiently — which can come with certain illnesses or old age. When we have metabolic issues we are sometimes left with the unhappy need to take supplements. Taking supplements shouldn't be necessary for a normal, healthy person. But it is a good alternative when, for some reason, our bodies are not metabolizing nutrients properly. Taking your physician's advice seriously if or when you encounter any problems is essential.

So we can see that some meat — with its unavoidable cholesterol and saturated fat — is required in your diet. Now let me help you to understand why both the cholesterol and saturated fat have been considered by many knowledgeable people to be a problem.

What I'm going to give you in the following description is greatly over-simplified and leaves out a whole bunch of detail. I do want to say that I am particularly grateful to a few expert sources: The University of Waterloo,[2] Dr. Peter Attia,[3] and Lyle McDonald's Body Recomposition website (www.bodyrecomposition. com).[4] These made a complex process much more understandable to this layperson! You should note also that the description will probably sound very sequential, as if only one thing happens in your body at a time. This is, of course, incorrect but it helps to explain it that way.

Okay, let's dive in.

Fat and Cholesterol in your Meal

Fats and cholesterol bounce around quite a bit in your body. The fats in a meal are broken down into fatty acids in the small intestine, packaged together with the cholesterol in the meal (cholesterol is a different kind of fat) into a form of lipoprotein called chylomicrons, and delivered directly into the blood stream. All this "packaging" has to happen because fat and water don't mix so the fats cannot travel through the blood without a protein "boat." The fats are extracted from the chylomicrons and absorbed by the muscles, organs, and fat cells. The cholesterol is left behind and is absorbed by the liver.

Now the liver has taken delivery of some cholesterol.

Carbohydrates in your Meal

In the meantime the carbohydrates you ate in that same meal are digested into sugars including glucose and fructose. The glucose enters the bloodstream and is available as energy for cells. The fat cells lock their fat away in the presence of the sugar and resulting insulin, making the glucose the only energy source. Any glucose not taken up by cells is returned to the liver. Fructose, on the other hand, goes directly to the liver where it is processed. The liver has to do something with all that energy from glucose and fructose so it first replenishes the glycogen (back up supply of quick energy) and then converts the rest into more triglycerides (fat).

If the amount of cholesterol and fat available are insufficient the liver (and most other body cells) will create them. The bulk of cholesterol used by the normal body is created by the liver. So the liver now has cholesterol (possibly both eaten and created) along with a new supply of triglycerides (fat) to handle.

Handling means packaging both into a different kind of lipoproteins called VLDL (Very Low Density Lipoproteins) and delivering them into the blood stream.

Protein in your Meal

Proteins (both animal and plant) are broken down into amino acids in the small intestine.

The amino acids go directly to the poor, overworked liver, then into the blood stream from where they are absorbed into the body tissues as needed. Every single cell in the body is constructed of protein and the amino acids are combined to rebuild or create that protein. The protein in body cells is always in a state of deterioration and restoration which is why we have to keep eating protein. Amino acids derived from protein are the body's energy source of last resort as they will be converted into glucose or even fatty acids when necessary.

VLDL and LDL cholesterol

In the bloodstream VLDL first delivers the new supply of triglycerides to the muscles, organs as needed, excess into fat cells. Left containing largely cholesterol, the VLDL is then transformed into a slimmer, trimmer LDL which begins distributing needed cholesterol to the body cells. Inevitably, there is some left over in this process.

HDL Cholesterol

To accommodate the left-over the liver also manufactures and delivers another lipoprotein call HDL to the bloodstream. Among other things HDL's job is to vacuum up the residue and return it to the liver. Some of the excess cholesterol will be excreted from the body as waste and the balance is recycled.

This sounds like a nice smooth progression so what causes it to breakdown? How does all that relate to cardiovascular disease? A lot of factors create potential for problems and things just get all mucked up. You have some genetic issues, conditions throughout the body create inflammation, the fats in your diet are bad fats, excess carbohydrate consumption creates excess blood glucose and insulin along with excess body fat and a fatty liver, the list goes on.

In the end it is agreed by experts that the amount and condition of LDL in your blood is the big problem in cardiovascular disease. And as we have seen, inflammation in the blood vessel walls makes them susceptible to absorbing

LDL. Thus the trouble starts:

- Excess sugar in the blood coats protein in the blood vessels walls creating advanced glycation end products (AGEs) which damage the vessel walls.

- The excess sugar can join together with LDL cholesterol particles in the blood, also creating AGEs, creating more inflammation, and making the LDL more easily deposited within blood vessel walls.

- And finally, once LDL has become glycated it is no longer recognized by the LDL receptor on cell surfaces, meaning that it can't offload the cholesterol and will continue bouncing up against the walls of the damaged blood vessel. Eventually LDL particles stick and can be absorbed into the vessel walls.

- And when that happens, your immune system leaps forward to heal the damage—first blood will clot to stop bleeding, then more inflammation occurs, and finally plaque builds up to seal over the damage. And this can happens over and over again until the plaque buildup can actually block the flow of blood in the vessel creating a myriad of potential problems.

A typical measure in your "lipid profile" ordered by your doctor at your annual physical is the amount of cholesterol in the LDL particles, a figure that is usually calculated rather than directly measured. However it appears now that the most important measure of cardiovascular risk is the actual number of LDL particles in your blood rather than the amount of cholesterol being carried. This makes sense to a reasonable mind since the more LDL particles banging up against an inflamed vessel wall, the more LDL is likely to stick and become embedded.

There is an amount of cholesterol needing delivery in your body and there is just so much room in a particle. The more triglycerides taking up space, the less space for cholesterol. Consequently, more particles are needed to accommodate the cholesterol and the more particles, the greater the risk.

Whether you know the number of LDL particles in your blood or not, I can tell you how you personally can impact that number and lower your risk. The amount of VLDL is the real driver because that determines how much LDL there will be, regardless of its structure.

Your LDL left the liver as VLDL and was transformed into LDL after dropping off most of the triglycerides created from excess sugar and fructose. Unless you have some sort of genetic abnormality, your diet is determining the amount of fat (from sugar and fructose) in need of transport—the more that needs to be transported, the more LDL particles ultimately created.

It took almost 100 years from the advent of Crisco, the very first partially hydrogenated oil, for the dangers to be recognized and then publically accepted by the USDA. The same thing is going on now around grain. Happily, the USDA now believes grain should be whole and not processed refined grain. Nonetheless, perhaps in the interest of not taking all the manufacturers to their economic knees, the current USDA recommendation is that "half" of daily grain eaten should be "whole grain." For a very long time the USDA and a portion of the healthcare community have been sticking it out that dietary cholesterol and saturated fat, to the exclusion of all else, is the cause of cardiovascular disease. Cholesterol as an official "nutrient of concern" appears now to be on its way out, leaving dietary saturated fat as the bad guy.

Lyle McDonald puts the issue of fat in context on his Body Recomposition website:

> The overall impact of any fat (including saturated fats) on health risk depends on the context of their intake. In one context (e.g. low fruit/vegetable/anti-oxidant intake, high stress, inactivity, high body fat, excessive total energy intake), a high saturated fat intake may be exceedingly harmful. In a different context (e.g. high fruit/vegetable intake, low stress, high activity, low body fat, appropriate energy intake), they may have no effect.[5]

But even that may not always be true. Consider the traditional diet of the Inuit Eskimos, which didn't include much in the way of fruits and vegetables. Not many plants grow in ice; the Inuit once subsisted almost entirely on animals and fish. The western diet provides vitamin C from fruits and vegetables. And the absence of vitamin C creates scurvy, a connective tissue disease. Surprisingly vitamin C really is available in the meat if eaten raw or minimally cooked. And calcium is also available, particularly in fish and seafood with soft, edible bones. So everything these Eskimos needed for a healthy diet is included in what appears to us as a very restricted and troublesome diet.

Actually the largest element in the Inuit diet was fat, but not the same kind of fat that we Americans find in our meat. Eric Dewailly, a professor at Laval University in Quebec, explained this fact in a Discover Magazine report on the "Inuit Paradox"—

> Wild animals that range freely and eat what nature intended … have fat that is far more healthful. Less of their fat is saturated, and more of it is in the monounsaturated form (like olive oil). What's more, cold-water fishes and sea mammals are particularly rich in polyunsaturated fats called n-3fatty acids or omega-3 fatty acids. These fats appear to benefit the heart and vascular system. But the polyunsaturated fats in most Americans' diets are the omega-6 fatty acids supplied by vegetable oils. By contrast, whale blubber consists of 70 percent monounsaturated fat and close to 30 percent omega-3s.[6]

So it's probably not cholesterol and fat per se but rather the sources of cholesterol and fat along with the sugar intensive processed foods that are the problems in your diet. The American diet may have created chronic inflammation and already wreaked havoc on your blood vessels, which changes the picture. So, yes, the amount of inflammation, fructose/glucose generated fat, number of LDL particles, and consequent plaque all matter—a lot.

Even if you haven't seen a doctor in many years, you do know what you have been eating. Assume there has been damage to your cardiovascular system and eat accordingly—which means, beyond following the other guidelines in this book, using judgment in eating meat and doing your best to make sure that meat is from animals that "range freely and eat what nature intended." While there is bountiful nutrition in meat and fish, there is no nutritional reason to consume cholesterol and saturated fat to excess when your cardiovascular system is already at risk. Two to three servings of meat or fish per week along with cheese, eggs, and milk can meet your B12 and omega-3 needs. That, plus all of the plant food in your diet meets your protein needs as well.

There are certainly many risk factors for your vascular system that are not food-related. Your liver may be "working overtime" (as my friend's doctor told her recently). Some inherit or for some other reason have genetic abnormalities that cause the system to go awry no matter what they do. This book does not provide medical advice on treatment of a damaged cardiovascular system. That is the job of your doctor. But it does provide commonsense guidance on how to avoid creating further damage. Preventing damage and avoiding further damage is essentially the same thing.

Nothing you can do will change your genetics. But you can control your diet and environment and minimize your risk for cardiovascular disease.

....

END NOTES

1   Harvard Medical School, "Listing of Vitamins," Harvard Health Publications & Newsweek Magazine collaboration on "Diet & Carbs" (January 19, 2004). Online at: http://www.health.harvard.edu/newsweek/ Listing_of_vitamins.htm (accessed December 17, 2014).

2   Michael Palmer, "Cholesterol Transport" Lecture notes for course on Human Metabolism, University of Waterloo. Online at: http://watcut. uwaterloo.ca/webnotes/Metabolism/cholesterolTransport.html (accessed February 27, 2014). See also Michael Palmer, "Digestion and uptake of dietary triacylglycerol," Lecture notes for course on Human Metabolism, University of Waterloo. Online at: http://watcut.uwaterloo.ca/webnotes/ Metabolism/fatTagDigestion.html (accessed February 27, 2014). For Dr. Palmer's faculty biography, see http://science.uwaterloo.ca/~mpalmer/.

3   Peter Attia, "The Straight Dope on Cholesterol – Part V," The Eating Academy blog (May 23, 2012). Online at: http://eatingacademy.com/ nutrition/the-straight-dope-on-cholesterol-part-v (accessed February 27, 2014). See also Peter Attia, "The Straight Dope on Cholesterol – Part VII," The Eating Academy blog (June 13, 2012). Online at: http:// eatingacademy.com/nutrition/the-straight-dope-on-cholesterol-part-vii (accessed February 27, 2014).

4   Lyle McDonald, "A Primer on Nutrition – Part 2," Body Recomposition website (October 2009). Online at: http://www.bodyrecomposition.com/ nutrition/a-primer-on-nutrition-part-2.html (accessed March 1, 2014).

[5]   Lyle McDonald, "A Primer on Dietary Fats – Part 2," Body Recomposition website (May 2009). Online at: http://www.bodyrecomposition.com/nutrition/a-primer-on-dietary-fats-part-2.html/ (accessed March 1, 2014).

[6]   Patricia Gadsby and Leon Steele, "The Inuit Paradox: How can people who gorge on fat and rarely see a vegetable be healthier than we are?" Discover Magazine (October 1, 2004). Online at: http://discovermagazine.com/2004/oct/inuit-paradox#.Ub3o5tic3Kc (accessed February 27, 2014).

CHAPTER ELEVEN

Vitamins, Minerals, and All

Vitamins (such as vitamin E and C), minerals (like calcium and iron), and other nutrients are required to support body structure, to regulate the body's process of converting food into energy (metabolism), and to fight back against inflammation. This stuff shows up in the food we eat. Check out these key facts about the vital nutrients our body needs:

- So far there are at least 25 named vitamins and minerals, heaven only knows how many antioxidants, phytonutrients and flavonoids, some 5000 or more enzymes, and a pile of fatty and amino acids required for the operation of the human body. (Researchers probably identified new ones yesterday!) With the exception of some enzymes, these are elements that must or should be consumed in food.

- All of the nutrients needed by the body can be found in the spectrum of food including protein, fats, and carbohydrates, with one absolute and two probable exceptions:

  - Vitamin B12 is manufactured by bacteria working on cobalt found in good earth and water. Plants take up the cobalt and animals/fish eat the plants. From a practical perspective B12 is only available in animal protein like meat, fish, eggs, and milk. Even then, the meat in animals can be B12 deficient if those animals are feeding on plants living in soil deficient in cobalt, a condition that is not uncommon in damaged soil. (Just another reason for avoiding chemical fertilizers and pesticides!)

- Remember that omega-3 fatty acids in any significant amounts are found in grass-fed meat and wild caught coldwater fish. In nature, fish feed either on each other or on the plants and algae that grow in the water. The only significant human food sources of vitamin D are fortified milk, butter, etc. and fatty fish such as salmon. Ideally, vitamin D is created by the interaction of sunlight with the cholesterol in our skin.

- There are thousands of phytonutrients (phyto meaning plant) found in low carbohydrates vegetables and fruits — those same vegetables that the average American doesn't eat many of. You cannot get all these in a pill.

- Vitamins A, D, E, and K are said to be "fat soluble," which means you need to eat them with some fat for them to be absorbed into and used by the body. If you eat these in natural food, that food always includes some fat. This explains why the instructions on the bottle of vitamins might say to "take with food." The body stores these vitamins in body fat and the liver and draws on them when required. The other vitamins (vitamins C, B series—not including B12) are water soluble and are not stored. That means we have to eat them every day and any excess we consume is washed out. Vitamin B12 is the exception, being water soluble but also being stored in the liver.

- According to the National Institutes of Health, the daily B12 requirement is 2.4 mcg of available B12.[1] Calculating on their tables, this amounts to the following:
    - 3.5 ounces of fish
    - over four 3 oz servings of top sirloin
    - about twenty 3 oz servings of chicken
    - five 8 ounce cups of milk
    - 5 cups plain yogurt
    - 5 servings of cheese
    - 10 eggs

- It is evident from this list that the most concentrated sources of B12 come from seafood, handy because they are also the best sources of omega-3. But from a practical perspective, the recommended 2.4 mcg of

B12 can be acquired from 2 eggs, 3 servings of cheese, and 2 cups of milk or yogurt. Both chicken and beef are excellent protein but very large amounts would be needed if each were the only source of B12 in your diet. For reasons described earlier, such large daily quantities of beef or chicken are not a good idea. Remember that your body stores B12 and then operates on that storage. So assuming your mother ate correctly, you started out life with a good supply. That means that a day without B12 can be compensated for tomorrow or the next week or even next month. Thus we don't actually need to eat meat every day.

· For most of us, especially the younger folks, all the nutrition we need can be found in a diverse diet of meat, fats, and carbohydrates. However a portion of us, particularly those who are growing older, find it harder to actually use the entire set of nutrients we need — even if we manage to eat them all. When this happens, nutritional supplements may be required. A medical practitioner or nutritionist is best equipped to advise on the issue of dietary supplements.

....

END NOTES

[1] Office of Dietary Supplements, "Dietary Supplement Fact Sheet: Vitamin B12," National Institutes of Health. Online at: http://ods.od.nih.gov/ factsheets/VitaminB12-HealthProfessional/ (accessed December 17, 2014).

CHAPTER TWELVE

Enzyme Deficiencies, Autoimmune Diseases, and Allergies

We eat food but our bodies don't (or shouldn't) absorb food directly. Instead enzymes are required to break that food down into nutrients. Enzymes aren't very sexy or particularly entertaining but they are absolutely critical. How many enzymes are there? According to Karen DeFelice, author of multiple books on enzymes, there may be millions because each has a specific and unique job in keeping our bodies functioning.[1]

Digestion involves the conversion of carbohydrates into glucose sugar, protein into amino acids, and fat into fatty acids. It takes place with the help of enzymes created by the body as well as enzymes naturally occurring in food itself. According to food enzyme researcher, Dr. Edward Howell, "Without enzymes, no activity at all would take place. Neither vitamins, minerals, or hormones can do any work — without enzymes."[2]

Actually there are three groups of enzymes. A unique set of metabolic enzymes operate within every cell of your body aiding in the amazingly complex processes required to keep you getting up every morning. Digestive enzymes created by the body break down food, allowing nutrients to be absorbed and used. Food enzymes are supplied by the food we eat. If the enzymes in food are diminished or missing (a condition that occurs when food is cooked), the digestive enzymes come in as a replacement.

Raw food only has enough enzymes to digest that particular food. For example, the enzymes in an apple are just enough for that one apple. When food is cooked above 118 degrees wet or 150 degrees dry, the enzymes are reduced or completely destroyed (depending on the level of heat), forcing enzymes created by the body to do double duty for digestion to complete.

If you are missing a particular enzyme, you will likely know it. Consider gluten, the protein in wheat, barley and rye that allows bread to rise and be fluffy. Gluten digestion requires protease enzymes to break it down into amino acids. Without that enzyme the gluten will not digest and severe digestive upset can result. Another example is lactose, the sugar in milk that requires the enzyme lactase to digest. Approximately 25% of adult Americans are lactose intolerant because their bodies do not create the lactase enzyme. Note that both of these examples include food that has been heated to high temperatures, effectively destroying the natural enzymes that came with the food and thus depending on enzymes created, or in these cases, not created by the body.

Enzyme deficiencies can be caused by a wide variety of things including genetics, pancreatic diseases (the pancreas makes most of the enzymes), inflammation in the digestive tract, chronic stress, and just plain aging, to name a few. Deficiency doesn't necessarily mean you have none of the enzyme, but you might just not have enough for a significant volume of a food. Note that there are likely many different enzymes required to digest any one food so it may not be easy to identify which one is missing.

Different from enzyme deficiencies are autoimmune diseases and allergies. There are people with autoimmune diseases like lupus, rheumatoid arthritis, and type 1 diabetes as examples. These diseases occur when the immune system, for some reason, attacks some part of the body. In lupus, the immune system attacks the body's tissues and organs. An allergy, on the other hand, is an immune response to something introduced from the outside like toxins or food.

Allergies vary in intensity but can be important sources of inflammation, occurring when the immune system mistakes a food element as harmful and attacks it. Symptoms can vary including things like nausea, cramping, diarrhea, hives, or swelling lips, tongue, or throat. At its worst an allergy can be life threatening, as is sometimes the case with peanuts and shellfish.

Celiac disease, caused by an allergic reaction to gluten in wheat, barley, and rye, is quite serious and those who have it should avoid all gluten. However, it appears now that some people have sensitivity to gluten that has not become celiac disease. These folks can handle a little gluten but will react to a lot. Chances are that this is an enzyme deficiency, but it is not always clear which enzyme is lacking since there are multiple enzymes involved.

My granddaughter had stomach problems all her young life — cramping, vomiting, and the like — but no test could uncover the cause. Finally, as I was doing the research for this book, her mother and I decided to do a test. As with many children, my granddaughter always had her hand in a cereal box. We removed eggs, milk, and anything with gluten from her diet and then added them back in, one at a time. She first recovered immediately and remained fine as we slowly added eggs and then milk back into her diet. Then we gave her cereal and almost immediately the old symptoms reared their ugly heads. She has had no problems since gluten was removed from her diet and, in fact, an occasional cracker causes no harm. A happy byproduct is that the reduction in sugar from wheat allowed her to lose weight.

I learned recently of a young woman with rheumatoid arthritis who was plagued with swelling ankles and feet along with persistent diarrhea. She blamed her medications. But she began researching and then adopted the Paleo diet which contains no grain or sugar. Both conditions disappeared as soon as she changed what she ate. The proof was in her wedding anniversary when she retrieved and ate left over wedding cake from her freezer. The next day her ankles and feet were swollen. Unfortunately she ate another piece and then missed work with diarrhea. We can't know, of course, whether it was the grain, the sugar, or both but at this point she doesn't really care because she feels really good.

In the case of lactose intolerance, the immune system is not in attack mode. Rather, as explained above, the body doesn't make the enzyme lactase required to digest the carbohydrate lactose in milk. So when my sister drank more than just a little regular cow's milk she got sick. She corrected that problem by drinking lactose-free milk. But she could have also supplemented with lactase, or given up milk entirely.

I have found no research that would definitively identify the prevalence of allergies. But the top eight most common allergens are clear: dairy, egg, wheat, soy, peanuts, tree nuts, fish and shellfish.[3] The first six are commonly found in processed food. If your body reacts negatively to a certain food, particularly if the reaction is persistent, you should seek help in locating and eliminating the source of the problem. Certainly it would be good to see your doctor. But if the tests don't find the source(s) of your allergic reaction or your pocketbook is limited, then you may have to ferret this out on your own.

If you have any of the symptoms described above and have no success with your doctor, the odds are that your body doesn't like something you are eating. The answer is not taking antacids or painkillers but rather first trying to find the cause and excluding it from your diet. Consider what you eat carefully and try to eliminate the most likely candidates—those you tend to eat the most. For example, if you are a big consumer of artificial sweeteners in drinks or food, stop consuming them for two weeks. The level of allergic reactions to aspartame in our population is pretty surprising. If aspartame is the cause your symptoms will likely disappear and then come roaring back when you drink your first diet soda.

Perhaps you eat lots of wheat products like bread, crackers, pasta, etc. Cut these foods out for a couple weeks and see what happens. If nothing changes then try eliminating dairy. On the other hand you may choose, as my daughter did, to cut out several of the usual suspects like dairy, wheat, and eggs all at one time, adding them back in one at a time to see if the trouble goes away and then returns.

It can be tricky uncovering the source of reactions to food, especially when the most common allergens are mixed up in processed food. This is just another good reason to avoid processed food! You will not get a good test if you don't consider the ingredients in all the food you eat. In my later chapter "Read the Label" I talk about how important it is to pay attention to the ingredients on things you buy. You can learn to identify some different ingredient names that might come from eggs or milk, or will actually be MSG (also a common allergen). And hiding out in the ingredients listed as "flavorings" can be mountains of chemicals you may also be reacting to.

A very few of you will be plagued with all the symptoms described above and none of the obvious eliminations work to resolve the problem. In this case you may be reacting to the content of multiple different carbohydrate foods and chemical additives all at the same time. Significant damage may have been done to your system and this is not going to be an easy fix.

Research done by Elaine Gottschall, biochemist, cell biologist, and author of Breaking the Vicious Cycle, looks at the complex relationships between food, the digestive system, and recovery, especially as it relates to autistic children but equally relevant to us all.[4] (You can read about Mrs. Gottschall at her website, http://www.breakingtheviciouscycle.info/.) There are several diets developed around her principles. Don't hesitate to use the Internet for help— just make sure the source you find is reputable and backed up by scientific research. And if you can afford it, find a medical doctor who also practices functional or holistic medicine.

Allergies and autoimmune conditions are a painful source of inflammation. And as you now know, chronic inflammation is hazardous to your health.

....

END NOTES

[1]   Karen DeFelice, "Fact Sheet on Enzymes," EnzymeStuff website. Online at: http://www.enzymestuff.com/faq.htm (accessed December 17, 2014). See also Karen DeFelice, Enzymes: Go With Your Gut: More Practical Guidelines For Digestive Enzymes (ThunderSnow Interactive, 2006).

[2]   "Interview with Dr. Edward Howell on Enzymes," Healthview Newsletter, R-Garden website. Online at: http://www.rgarden.com/55.html (accessed February 27, 2014).

[3]   "The Most Common Food Allergies: The Top 8," Eating With Food Allergies website. Online at: http://www.eatingwithfoodallergies.com/commonfoodallergies.html (accessed December 17, 2014).

[4]   Elaine Gottschall, Breaking the Vicious Cycle: Intestinal Health Through Diet (Kirkton Press, 1994).

CHAPTER THIRTEEN

What the Heck is Phytic Acid?

As if that starchy sugar thing with grain weren't enough, there is a further complication. It seems that grain, beans, and nuts/seeds are difficult for us humans to digest and this turns out to be important. So in order that you may understand the problem, let's begin with a discussion of plants and how they reproduce.

As all gardeners know, there is always a seed and the seed is always designed to allow for germination at just the right time. That is a unique point when the soil and air temperature, moisture, and light are just right for that plant. Phosphorus is a critical mineral in the development of a plant. Seeds store most of their phosphorus in the form of phytic acid. Phytic acid reaches out and latches onto most of the other minerals in the seed and inhibits the enzymes required to digest the nutrition in the seed. Thus, premature germination of the seed is avoided.

Now consider how we eat the plants. Sometimes we eat the product resulting from the germination, like lettuce, cauliflower, oranges, avocados, peppers, tomatoes, etc. By the time the plant matures and is ready to be eaten an enzyme called phytase has unlocked the phosphorous which, in turn, frees up the other minerals and enzymes. Only a small residue of phytic acid remains.

But sometimes we don't eat the plant itself but rather the next generation of seeds that the plant produces. This would be things like beans, nuts, and seeds such as pinto beans, almonds, and flax. In other words we are eating the seeds of future plants. Of course, those seeds are also chock full of nutrition, the very nutrition that would allow the plant to grow upon germination. But just as with the lettuce seed, the phytic acid in the outside layer of the bean/grain/nut seed locks up the minerals and inhibits the action of the enzymes, patiently waiting for the right time to germinate.

Of course, with beans and nuts we mean to eat the seed and not wait for another plant to grow. The Agriculture Research Service at the USDA provides the following explanation for phytic acid and grain, which is equally relevant for beans and nuts:

> Humans need minerals to stay healthy, and people rarely have phosphorus deficiencies. But cereals like rice store most phosphorus in the grain as phytic acid, which can't be digested by one-stomached animals like fish, chickens, pigs, and humans. It binds to minerals such as iron, calcium, magnesium, and zinc in the slightly acidic conditions in our intestines. Because phytic acid is poorly digested and used, the minerals it binds to are less available to our bodies.[1]

Here is the deal. The human body generally doesn't make digestive phytase so when the phytic acid needs phytase to break it down, the food just won't digest. And in addition to the minerals that are unavailable we also have (ahem) gastrointestinal discomfort. Almost all commercially farmed animals are fed grains and are thus susceptible to nutritional deficiencies, deficiencies met by adding supplements to their feed. Among those supplements would be the phytase enzyme to reduce phytic acid.

For people, the whole idea of minerals from food being "locked up" doesn't sound good, does it? This seems to be one of those good news/bad news things. Some reports warn about how bad it is, but others point out the good side. It turns out that both these views are right.

The good news about phytic acid is that it binds with and helps your body dispose of toxic heavy metals you may have been exposed to, metals like arsenic and lead. A healthy body has an answer to most problems and this is one of them. That residual phytic acid in vegetables is in there doing an important job. The bad news is that we Americans with our unbalanced diet eat too much grain, thus consuming too much phytic acid and consequently locking up a lot of other good minerals along with the bad. To make matters worse, legumes like beans and nuts, super good sources of protein and good fat, are also seeds and have the same issue with phytic acid.

We need those minerals and surely, one would think, there must be some way to fool Mother Nature and make her believe that now is the "right time" for germination (read: digestion). Yes, there is a way we can, to some degree, accomplish that very thing.

Consider the diet of the ancient Israelites in Bible times. Bread made from emmer wheat and barley was a staple of their diet. The phytic acid was there, but the difference was in the processing. They stone ground their grain and made sourdough bread daily. The fresh grinding maximized the available nutrients and avoided spoilage while the sourdough processing, lactic fermentation, released the phytic acid. They ate lentil stew with vegetables daily as well. Lentils have a lower level of phytic acid compared to many other legumes. The rest of their diet included good oil (olive); goat's milk, butter, and cheese; a small variety of vegetables; fruit like figs, pomegranates and grapes; and some occasional goat or sheep meat. In other words, every nutritional need was met on a very narrow diet and the phytic acid issues were minimized.

They accomplished this by using the resources that the good Lord provided without benefit of electricity, refrigeration, or scientific research. We can't say the same today. Commercial "scientific" research, too much of which looks for the cheapest and fastest way to do something without equal attention to consequences, has gotten us where we are today.

Look first at today's bread. Phytic acid is not a problem at all in products made from refined flour (ground up grain from which the outside layers of bran and germ have been removed). The phytic acid is in the outside layers of the grain along with most of the nutrition and fiber. So that bread largely contributes only sugar from the starch in the inside layer, the endosperm, and would be pretty useless nutritionally if the producer didn't add some back in at the behest of the USDA. The nutritional value and digestive problem are both handed off to the bran and germ that were ground off, sold for animal feed or sometimes packaged separately by the producer and sold at a premium. Special deal! No phytic acid, at least not in the bread. Plenty in the bran and germ.

The situation is different, obviously, with whole grain breads. All the nutrition is still there but not necessarily "available" due to the phytic acid. Just for clarity, the endosperm as the main source of starchy sugar is also still there.

So you can see this looks like a no-win deal. The refined flour bread is a loser nutritionally. And the whole grain can also be at least a partial loser if we don't break down the phytic acid and release the minerals. This is, fortunately, doable if you are making your own bread or can find someone to do it for you.

One alternative is bread made from sprouted grain flour, as the sprouting accomplishes the initial germination thus reducing a portion of the phytic acid. Whole grain sourdough bread is best because sourdough "starter," ideally a rye starter, accomplishes quite a phytic acid reduction. You can find sprouted grain bread in the organic freezer section of some stores. But while you will find lots of breads in the stores labeled as "sourdough" they are most often yeasted bread with a sour flavoring. Yeasted bread is much faster and thus much cheaper to make. Not much impact on the phytic acid.

I would like to tell you that you can get "real" sourdough at a bakery. But I have personally seen a bakery that buys their mix from somewhere else, plops it in the oven and bakes. Ask questions. Your best bet may be a home-baker who is willing to sell or a friend who likes you a lot. There are many books and websites providing detailed instructions on bread making if you would like to give it a try. You will find two things to be true. Making sourdough bread at home takes time, planning, and equipment—but the results are delicious!

The Nourished Kitchen website (www.nourishedkitchen.com) is a great resource for helping you understand what is required to make good sourdough bread, both the starter and the bread itself. My favorite is the challah bread but it is just one example of many.[2] I am not recommending this site above all others, but I do like how clearly it addresses the phytic acid issue and the respect shown for quality ingredients.

This brings us to all that other grain stuff like dry cereal, oatmeal, rice, cornmeal, tortilla chips, etc. Dry cereal has exactly the same issues as commercial breads, both refined and whole grain. Further, cereals are frequently processed at extreme heats and sometimes contain unhealthy ingredients including the ever-popular sugar. All that heat reduces vitamins, kills the enzymes, and makes no impact on the phytic acid. Think about that the next time you see a child carrying around a cereal box.

You can make an impact on oatmeal, grits, quinoa, and rice by soaking them before cooking, although the impact varies. I have seen no magic solution for pasta unless you or somebody else makes it with soaked or sprouted grain. There are lots of folks on the Internet happy to show you how to make your own pasta. All of these, however, take planning ahead and some of us are pretty adapted to whipping it off the shelf, quickly cooking it and plopping it on the table.

If you are concerned about the loss of mineral nutrients in your grains but don't have the time or resources to deal with the problem directly, then you have three choices. Search until you find a supplier who is willing to do the work, give up grain (this would be the Paleo way), or limit the amount of grain you eat in any form (bread or otherwise) while ensuring extra nutrition to compensate for the mineral loss.

I read somewhere once that it is the dose that makes the poison. This is true for fructose, for nitrites, and for grain. Keep the amount of whole grain in line (1/2 cup or 1 slice servings) and the rest of your healthy diet will compensate for the phytic acid just as it did for the Israelites. In the upcoming chapter on Grain, Potatoes, and Sugar, I recommend that you limit the combination of grain and potatoes to six servings per day.

This brings us to beans (legumes) and nuts, important contributors to protein in a good diet. Just as with grains, you can make a big impact on the digestibility and nutritional value of beans and nuts by soaking before cooking. My grandmother taught me to soak my beans overnight before cooking but she, like the Israelites, didn't know about phytic acid. She and my mother and just about everyone else thought we were just making the beans cook faster. So when somebody dreamed up quicker methods, many stopped overnight soaking.

We should get back to soaking. I find the web site Deep Roots at Home: Enriching the Soil of Your Life (http://www.deeprootsathome.com/) to have a splendid level of detail regarding soaking both grains and beans.[3] But there are many websites you might find helpful, so take a look! I also want to share my approach for treating both beans and nuts. While the appropriate amount of soaking time varies because the amount of acid and phytase (food enzyme) in each bean/nut varies, the following two recipes will be workable for most.

Tips on Bean Treatment

Cover dry beans with 4 times bean volume of water. Add two or so tablespoons of an acid medium like lemon or vinegar. Vinegar is obviously cheaper. Cover and soak at least overnight and up to 24 hours. If you soak over 12 hours then drain, rinse, add more water and acid and let the soaking continue. Generally speaking, the longer the soak the more phytic acid is reduced. When ready to cook then drain and rinse, add seasonings, meat if you have some, and broth (chicken or vegetable) and cook on low heat until done. Use your favorite recipe. The beans will, indeed, cook faster after soaking.

You will likely find some yucky looking scum on top of the soaking water; this is stuff you want to get rid of which explains the importance of draining and rinsing. Any scum that appears while cooking should also be strained off. Since you are going to cook the beans, the food enzymes will be gone after cooking. You will be depending on your own digestive enzymes to take up the slack.

Final point on beans. They all contain a combination of sugars that require a particular enzyme to digest and we humans don't usually have that enzyme either. So the sugars get digested by bacteria in the large intestine. The inevitable outcome of this bacterial activity is gas which can be both uncomfortable and embarrassing—except for small boys. This may or may not be a problem for you but my experience is that the soaking process can also be helpful in reducing that problem. To some degree the problem also occurs because the phytic acid is indigestible.

Tips on Nut Treatment

Cover raw nuts (almond, pecan, peanut, and walnut) with a substantial amount of lightly salted water – don't be stingy with the water as the nuts will soak up the liquid. Soak at least 7 hours in a warm spot like your microwave or oven (turned off), drain and rinse the nuts well, shaking off as much liquid as possible. Spread nuts evenly on a foil covered oven tray (minimize cleanup) and bake on the lowest temperature possible in your oven—ideally 150 degree but 170 degrees in mine and probably yours. Bake until dry and crisp; 12-24 hours, stirring every now and then. A taste test will tell you when they are done. Cool completely before storing. Delicious!

Commercial nuts at the grocery may say roasted but don't expect them to be soaked and slow roasted. And, in fact, these are not the nuts you want to use. The nuts should be raw. Do you remember why 150 degrees? Because that is the dry temperature above which the food enzymes begin to deteriorate. Since my oven won't go down to 150 I settle for 170 and enzyme deterioration. A dehydrator is an alternative.

I usually soak my nuts during the day and then roast them during the night when I don't need the oven for other purposes. According to Sally Fallon in Nourishing Traditions, properly roasted pecans and almonds will last for several months on the shelf in your pantry or on your kitchen counter—I usually have a couple handfuls a day so my nuts go pretty fast.[4] But walnuts should be stored in the refrigerator because the oil in walnuts is very susceptible to spoiling, roasted or not.

I may have spent more time researching phytic acid than on any other single nutritional element in this book. Eventually I reached the conclusion that there is too much nutrition in the seeds that we eat for us to avoid them. In reality anything that grew from a seed, that is to say all plants, will have some phytic acid but the foods with the greatest implications are those where we actually eat the seeds. Beans and nuts are very important sources of protein, vitamins, fiber, and good oils in a diet that minimizes meat and the negatives can be handled effectively by soaking and cooking properly. It isn't even hard.

The tougher issue is the grain because we Americans consume so much of it, already processed, off the shelf at the grocery store. Frankly the USDA did not do us a favor when they recommended eating up to 11 servings per day because we now have a difficult habit to break. You simply have to keep that number of servings to six, get a handle on what a serving actually is, and minimize that stuff you can't fix—most dry cereal and all those commercially processed foods made of grain including chips, pasta, pizza dough, and store bought bread.

So you now have two good reasons to manage grain in your diet—because of both sugar and phytic acid.

END NOTES

[1]   Agricultural Research Service of the United States Department of
       Agriculture, "New Rice Could Benefit Malnourished Populations,"
       Agricultural Research Magazine 50:9 (September 2002). Online at:
       http://www.ars.usda.gov/is/AR/archive/sep02/rice0902.htm (accessed
       December 17, 2014).

[2]   Jenny McGruther, "A Recipe: Sourdough Challah with Poppy Seeds"
       Nourished Kitchen website (November 29, 2011). Online at: http://
       nourishedkitchen.com/whole-wheat-sourdough-challah/ (accessed
       December 17, 2014).

[3]   "Soaking Beans and Grains ~ ByeBye Phytic Acid and Beano," Deep
       Roots at Home website (January 7, 2013). Online at: http://www.
       deeprootsathome.com/soaking-beans-and-grains-byebye-phytic-acid-and-
       beano/ (accessed February 27, 2014).

[4]   See Sally Fallon with Mary G. Enig, Nourishing Traditions: The
       Cookbook that Challenges Politically Correct Nutrition and the Diet
       Dictocrats (Washington, DC: New Trends Publishing, Inc., 2001).

CHAPTER FOURTEEN

Fats and Oils

Lowering dietary omega-6 fat means cooking primarily with olive oil and limiting processed foods to those made with olive oil, canola oil, or high-oleic oils. The top three contributors of omega-6 fat in the diet are soybean oil, cottonseed oil and corn oil, plus foods made with these oils (such as margarines, salad dressings and mayonnaise).

When cooking and making food purchases, there are a few key tips to keep in mind related to fats and oils:

1. Avoid anything advertised as "reduced fat." This is very popular labeling, sometimes even when the food didn't have fat in it in the first place. When the fat is removed the manufacturer has to put something else in as a substitute and that something usually amounts to sugar and/or some other filler. Fillers rarely add nutrition (and sugar certainly doesn't).

2. Make extra virgin olive oil (EVOO) your cooking and salad oil of choice. EVOO has the highest level of monounsaturated fat, and has higher levels of antioxidants and anti-inflammatory properties. Ideally the bottle label of extra virgin olive oil would say cold pressed—which means it was extracted without heat. But if cold pressed is not an option, then settle for plain old EVOO. But always go extra-virgin. While extra virgin olive oil will likely cost more than other oils, you shouldn't be frying with it. So you won't be using that much. The cooking temperature of EVOO should be below 350 degrees, usually medium on your range top.

3. You can make your own salad dressings with EVOO. Red wine vinegar, EVOO and maybe an optional touch of lemon is a fine, simple, and inexpensive alternative. But if this is not an option, read the label on everything and try to avoid those products that include soybean, cottonseed, or corn oil and, of course, partially hydrogenated oil.

If your pocket book will allow it, there are other non-grain specialty oils tasty for dressings. Most, however, are susceptible to oxidation and rancidity, which means they should be permanently stored in the refrigerator.

Actually it is very difficult to find processed foods containing only olive oil or canola oil although you may find some that say "soybean oil, corn oil, or canola oil," as an example. Given that soybean and corn oils may be the cheapest for the manufacturer (because of heavy government subsidies on those crops), canola is not likely to be the oil of choice but it looks good on the label.

Hain Pure Foods brand and WholeFoods 365 both produce a canola mayonnaise made with expeller pressed canola oil, a good choice. There may be others. There are recipes out there for making mayo at home; seek them out if you are so inclined. But note that plain whole (full fat) yogurt with a little flavoring is an excellent substitute for mayonnaise.

Somehow children (and adults) in our society have gotten very attached to ranch dressing. Making your ranch dressing homemade with healthy ingredients would be the best route—something you can easily find out how to do online. However, if you aren't making your own and can't get a raw vegetable into that child's mouth without first dipping it in store bought ranch dressing, then just do the best you can. The vegetables are very important.

4. If you insist on frying, then use refined canola like you find in the store and keep the temperature below 400 degrees. While canola is usually heat-processed, not the best, it does have a large percentage of monounsaturated oil and an excellent ratio of omega-6 to omega-3. Keep your canola refrigerated. Keep all your oils sealed and, except for olive and coconut, refrigerated or they can oxidize and become rancid.

You may be wondering about peanut oil, which obviously isn't made from grain. Technically peanuts are a legume (bean). Although refined peanut oil has a smoke point nearer to canola, it has no omega-3 and a ton of omega-6. Refined canola has the highest smoke point of all and should be your choice if you simply must fry.

The smoke point of oil is very important. Once the oil begins to smoke, the creation of trans-fats begins. Avoid smoking oils. Avoid any products that contain hydrogenated oil of any kind. Maybe I have mentioned that already!

5. When you can, cook at home. Most commercial products made with flour will include the oils I have suggested you avoid. From a health perspective, the best option is to cook your own food in your own kitchen. It takes time, but it is well worth it. Make the lifestyle decision, which in this case is also a health decision!

CHAPTER FIFTEEN

Grain, Potatoes, and Sugar

I'm sure you have gotten this point already but it is worth repeating. The big three foods containing carbohydrate for most Americans are grains, potatoes, and table sugar. Together they are the source of too darn much "sugar" in our diets, responsible for a lot of extra pounds attached to our bodies as well as the chronic health conditions often associated with those pounds. But because I know you like them (a lot) my goal here is to help you include them in your diet with minimal nutritional consequences. A lot of this is about the wisdom of practicing balance and good habits.

Grain

There are multiple grain varieties growing in the US and across the world, all significant sources of sugar in the form of starch. Certainly some of this grain is purchased whole and cooked at home. But the grains most often seen in your supermarket are wheat, oats, rice, and corn — all commonly ground up into flour and commercially processed into stuff like bread, crackers, pasta, pretzels, cereal, cookies and cakes, pie crust, chips, and tortillas. The list is endless, displayed in sacks and boxes along the shelves in the middle aisles of your grocery.

As mentioned before, at one time these products were called "refined" because the healthy parts of the grain were missing. Typically some of the missing nutrients were then added back in (chemically) and the products were thus called "enriched." These days some portion of the ground up grain is often whole grain, meaning that more of the healthy parts are still present. This is good news, sort of.

Good news because more nutrients are available. The bad news is that it is still grain ground-up into flour; thus the award winner for delivering sugar into your bloodstream at warp speed. This wouldn't be so bad if you weren't eating so much of it but, repeating myself I know, these commercially processed products make up a huge portion of the typical American diet. When we think grain most of us first imagine bread or cereal, but grain also hides out in places we least expect such as starchy fillers in most commercial salad dressings, ketchup, sauces, etc. So you can actually see the prevalence of processed grain just by looking at the number of grocery store aisles committed to these products and the contents of grocery carts in the checkout line. And it can get tricky, this whole grain thing. When you are searching for whole grain, don't be fooled by brown bread and crackers or the words "whole wheat" on the package. In the commercial world of additives it isn't difficult to color something brown. Read the ingredient list. "Whole wheat" does not necessarily mean "whole grain" and the ingredient list will tell the tale. You might not even be getting the extra nutrition promised with "whole grain."

Potatoes

Potatoes are very nutritious but, as we've already seen, they are also just packed with sugar in the form of starch. Again, this wouldn't be so bad if it weren't for French fries and potato chips. Certainly most fast food restaurant meals come with a substantial pile of fries and most of us eat them, sometimes even getting a double order. Oh my goodness, I don't even want to think how many greasy, salty French fries I have eaten over the years. Potato chips are extremely popular too, available in an ever growing number of chemically added flavors. So if you can't get to your favorite burger joint you can always substitute a nice bag of potato chips.

In appropriate portions potatoes are perfectly okay for a non-diabetic. But note that a serving size is a small red potato and think about how this compares to the amount you typically eat. French fried sweet potatoes grow more popular, operating on the theory that sweet potatoes are "healthier" than white potatoes. As with all food, white and sweet potatoes have significant nutritional value, albeit in different combinations. But what these potatoes most have in common is a lot of starch. So again, an excess of starch is problematic for your waistline and overall health.

Sugar

That white stuff in the sugar bowl on your table (along with brown sugar which is just white sugar colored with molasses) is simple processed sugar (sucrose) likely made from sugar cane or beets. About half of this sugar is glucose, immediately available for the body to burn for energy but bringing absolutely no nutritive value, high levels of acid, and a burst of blood sugar.

The balance of the sugar is fructose which is usually converted to body fat. Natural unrefined sugar sources such as honey and maple syrup also digest quickly but at least they do have a small complement of vitamins and minerals, are less acidic, and you don't eat such big amounts.

So this is just straight sugar, which isn't starch but is the most significant food additive in the typical American's diet besides salt. I'm talking about the sugar that is dumped into everything from soft drinks and "sports" beverages, to processed breakfast foods and snack bars, to condiments like barbecue sauce and ketchup. Don't be fooled by an ingredient list that lists high fructose corn syrup because HFCS is still sugar.

There is even bottled sugar. The shelves of pancake syrup at the store are tall and wide. And every bottle will include some form of sugar including high fructose corn syrup, usually as the first ingredient on the ingredient list. This is the same high fructose corn syrup mentioned above. Just remember the Israelites. They reduced fruit to syrup for sweetener because, in those days, nobody had yet dream up white, refined sugar or high fructose corn syrup.

Over time commercial food manufacturers have searched diligently for ways to sweeten without sugar, with mixed success. Aspartame and other "sugar free," chemically created sweeteners are also high acid with no nutrition. And sometimes they taste weird. The current best-choice sweetener seems to be Stevia. I have used Stevia on rare occasions. But since every "sugar free" sweetener has been found to be problematic sooner or later for one reason or another, I hesitate to call anything "safe."

And I should point out that, in baking volume, these products really aren't sugar free. In baking a sugar substitute needs to contribute not just the taste but also the body and texture of real sugar. In order to accomplish that with an artificial sweetener they have to add back in some form of sugar; sounds ridiculous I know. The amount of sweetener in one of those ½ tsp coffee sized packets is less than one carb. But multiply that by 94 to get a cup and you've got yourself some real sugar, no longer sugar free.

Overconsumption of sugar, whether from starches or out of a sugar bowl, is linked to cardiovascular disease, fatty liver disease, high blood pressure, type 2 diabetes, and kidney disease. I may have mentioned these before. And get this: recent studies have shown that sugar addiction leads to a "craving, tolerance, and withdrawal" pattern that is similar to hard drugs like cocaine and heroin![1] That craving and withdrawal phenomena exists even when artificial sweeteners are substituted for real sugar. It is a taste thing.

The truth of the matter is that Americans consume an average of 130 lbs. of straight sugar per year, more than enough to do major damage to our health.[2] There is so much added sugar in much of the food we buy that we really have to make an effort to reduce our intake. This should help. Large quantities of sugar almost invariably arrive in foods made from grain. The less processed grain in your diet, the less sugar likely to be eaten as a natural course.

How Much Starch is Okay?

The main trick to keeping grain, potatoes, and sugar in your diet is reducing the number and size of servings. Limit yourself to more than six servings of starch (grain and potatoes) per day, including snacks. Minimize anything processed, packaged into a box or sack, and sold in a store. Special, desert-like treats made at home, stuff like Aunt Mildred's famous coconut cream pie or mom's double chocolate chip cookies, should be occasional treats, not daily menu items.

As important as the number of servings is the size of servings. A substantial pile of French fries is easily six servings. And when it comes to processed foods like pasta which require cooking, the serving size on the label may be pretty useless and misleading. The amount that arrives on your plate is what matters. The following serving size examples may surprise you.

- A serving of rice, pasta, and oatmeal is ½ cup cooked (which isn't much).

- A serving of bread is one (not two) slices

- A serving of chips or crackers is usually 15

- A serving of cold cereal is usually ½ to ¾ cup.

- One pancake about the size of a compact disc is one serving.

- One small potato is a serving.

Get out your measuring cup (or compact disc) and measure out a few of these. To be honest, when I saw how small a serving of cold cereal was, I quickly decided it wasn't worth the effort. I stick to eggs. But if it just has to be cereal, you measure a time or two and then place the food on the plate or bowl, until you can measure by sight. Many people including children eat as much as three times that amount in a meal or snack.

Warning: Kids get hungry. Lots of children besides my granddaughter like to walk around with their hands in a cereal box. Just remember that most the cereals on the grocery shelves are extruded with high heat to get those cute little shapes and they really contain little other than sugar. If you are feeding your children cereal, find one that is whole grain without added sugar and then allow cereal (in the appropriate portion size) in no more than one meal or snack a day. Need I mention the fruit and milk? Keep a sack of blueberries in the freezer and toss in a handful. And stock your pantry and fridge with healthier snacks.

Not long ago I ate dinner at a popular Italian restaurant and watched a rotund gentleman at a nearby table attack a platter of spaghetti (along with a basket of bread) that should have fed the whole table. I might bet big money that someone in your family will eat as much as four or five cups of pasta with spaghetti sauce. Again, how many servings are in that nice, big bowl of cereal you eat every morning? How many and what size are the pancakes you ate recently? If you can't control serving sizes then avoid the food. Eat more vegetables; you can have all of those you want.

I can remember a time when I would pile up on the couch and watch a football game with a full box of Cheez-Its. And at the end of the game that box would probably be empty. I looked at that size Cheez-it box yesterday and found there to be (drum roll, please) 19 servings. This extraordinary amount of sugar contributed, no doubt, to my current diabetes. So, fair warning, don't hand your child (or yourself) a box or sack of anything. Dole out a serving if you choose to eat them. And don't have sacks of chips or pretzels in your house that include any of the best-avoided oils.

Many a meal, such as most Mexican entrees, will include several starches. The taco shell is already one grain serving. If you add an enchilada, it will be wrapped in another serving (or two). Two or more servings might be rice (1/2 cup) and beans (1/2 cup). In my experience the amount of rice and beans on your place is likely more. While beans are an excellent source of protein and other nutrients, they are also full of starch. Complicate this by eating a half basket or so of tortilla chips before the real meal even arrives. Wow!

That Mexican meal can easily cause high blood sugar in even the best of metabolism. A taco or an enchilada alone piled high with meat, lettuce, cheese, sour cream, salsa, etc. with a ½ cup serving of beans and a side salad is actually a complete and nutritious meal with a good proportion of protein, starch, vegetables, and fiber. Leave the rest for tomorrow.

The serving size of cornbread, cake, cookie, or any other sweet should about two inches; significantly smaller than you are used to eating. This brings us to the most offensive (as far as I'm concerned) of the processed grain/sugar products — Pop Tarts or Twinkies and that entire genre of grocery store sweets designed to fit nicely into a small child's hand — advertised with abandon and also on the shelves of every convenience store and service station. The touted "one serving of fruit" included in the Pop Tart turned to pure sugar and lost its nutritional value back at the manufacturing facility, if there was ever actually any fruit there in the first place. Just because it tastes like blueberries doesn't necessarily mean blueberries are actually in there.

There are people in this world who grind their own grain, soak the grain, and make their own bread or pasta or tortillas. Some use a sourdough starter to do the same. Consequently they are using the freshest ingredients and choosing their own oils. They are avoiding the myriad of preservatives and additives found in commercial products and maximizing the available nutrition in the food. This is a good thing as the soaking and sour dough options minimize the issues with phytic acid discussed a couple chapters back. However, whether making at home or buying at the store, the sugar is still there and it still counts.

Prevent Hunger

The second important trick to keeping starches in your diet is preventing hunger. Not long ago I walked into the OVI food pantry. One of our volunteers was scanning a USDA inventory list taped to a refrigerator, clutching a potato chip sack with one hand and shoveling chips into her mouth with the other. "I am starving," she said when she saw me. "That salad I had before I came didn't last very long." There is a reason for that!

An otherwise healthy pile of vegetables and a not-so-healthy sack of potato chips will both digest pretty quickly and hunger will soon follow. While there won't be much blood sugar impact from the salad, there will be a ton from the chips. In both cases, however, the hunger will return quickly. Protein and the accompanying fat like meat, cheese, eggs, beans, nuts, sour cream, etc. digest very slowly and make a great, more filling cover for a salad. Make the salad dressing oil-based, like red wine vinegar and olive oil, with no carbs in the mix. Combining meat and fat into a meal or a snack has two advantages: slowing the blood sugar increase and preventing hunger. Hunger is the enemy of healthy weight.

Repeating, carbohydrates in a meal should always be accompanied by protein and fat. A well constructed meal does not have to be complicated, but it should be filling. If you find yourself hungry in an hour or two, then there was not enough fat in the meal. Snacks should either be protein/fat based (hardboiled eggs, cheese, nuts) or be combinations as well. A good combination example would be slices of apple or a few crackers with peanut butter or cheese.

Can a carbohydrate alone be a good snack? A piece of fruit or some vegetables are both healthy, low calorie snacks, particularly for children who are always hungry. But any processed carbohydrate of the grain and chip variety will be high calorie and not very satisfying long term. Try to save your (unprocessed, wholefood) starch servings for meals.

Something as simple as a bean dip (you can make your own) or ranch dip helps to balance when eating tortilla chips or sliced vegetables. Guacamole (avocado) dip is also excellent and very satisfying. Be reasonable here: a tablespoon of dip and six or eight chips is about right for a snack; it's not a meal. Be sure to read the label carefully if you did not make the chips yourself. A proper tortilla chip will include only corn, lime, and water with maybe a little salt, absolutely no added oil, and it will naturally include plenty of fiber. Again, fiber and protein both help shield the starchy carbohydrates in food from rapid digestion.

In Summary

Limit yourself to six servings of starch (potatoes and grain) per day. Minimize processed grains and potatoes of any kind. Whenever possible, combine protein, fat, a little starch, and vegetables together in a meal. Try always to include a protein/fat in a snack. You will need to eat more vegetables to take the place of the starches you are removing from your diet.

....

END NOTES

1   James J. DiNicolantonio and Sean C. Lucan, "Sugar Season: It's Everywhere, and Addictive," New York Times (December 22, 2014). Online at: http://www.nytimes.com/2014/12/23/opinion/sugar-season-its-everywhere-and-addictive.html&assetType=opinion&_r=0 (accessed January 6, 2015). See also Table 1 in James J. DiNicolantonio and Sean C. Lucan, "The wrong white crystals: not salt but sugar as aetiological in hypertension and cardiometabolic disease," Open Heart (2014): 5. Online at: http://openheart.bmj.com/content/1/1/e000167.full.pdf+html (accessed April 23, 2015). In addition, DiNicolantonio and Lucan cite recent studies that "suggest intakes in the US population anywhere from 77 to 152 lbs of sugar per year" (4).

2   See Alice G. Walton, "How Much Sugar Are Americans Eating?" Forbes Online (August 30, 2012). Online at: http://www.forbes.com/sites/alicegwalton/2012/08/30/how-much-sugar-are-americans-eating-infographic/ (accessed December 17, 2014). Estimates of sugar

consumption vary widely due to the inherently difficult task of measuring it across a broad population. For example, a recent New York Times article noted that the USDA has reduced its official estimates of per capita sugar consumption [see Stephanie Strom, "U.S. Cuts Estimate of Sugar Intake," New York Times (October 26, 2012). Online at: http://www.nytimes.com/2012/10/27/business/us-cuts-estimate-of-sugar-intake-of-typical-american.html?pagewanted=all&_r=0 (accessed January 6, 2015)]. Yet DiNicolantonio and Lucan's citation of recent studies that "suggest intakes in the US population anywhere from 77 to 152 lbs of sugar per year" (DiNicolantonio and Lucan, "The wrong white crystals," 5), puts Walton's estimate of 130 lbs. well within range.

CHAPTER SIXTEEN

Milk and Milk Products

Milk or No Milk?

Technically the USDA's interest in milk appears to be largely associated with calcium and vitamin D fortification due to historical deficiencies—deficiencies usually occur when we don't eat what we should. Milk is considered by many Americans to be our primary source of calcium and the dairy industry helps that by adding extra calcium.

Milk is the only animal product that contains a carbohydrate. The carb in milk is called lactose. Lactose requires the enzyme lactase for digestion and lactase is made in the small intestine. The typical human baby's body makes lactase as long as he is fed milk but over time, the body simply slows down and frequently stops making lactase altogether. Thus, a good percentage of the world population becomes lactose intolerant after infancy and gets its calcium from plant sources. (So regardless of what the milk industry or the USDA says, there are other good calcium sources besides milk.)

If you are eating the proper amount/diversity of green vegetables and fruit, you can get all the calcium you need. But it may require some planning. Note, however, that milk-based (particularly whole milk-based) products are among the few significant dietary sources of vitamin D. Further, milk and all milk products are excellent low cost sources of protein and vitamin B12. So, if you are not lactose intolerant, there are good, cost-effective reasons to consume milk and milk products that have nothing to do with calcium.

Expert estimates of vitamin D deficiency vary markedly but according to the Scientific American, 75% of Americans are deficient in vitamin D.[1] Your body can't use the calcium you eat—calcium is a major component of your bones—

if it doesn't also have vitamin D. Thus, a vitamin D deficiency is critical. So remember that milk fat is one of the few food sources of vitamin D.[2]

The problem with milk has to do with spoiling. The perfect milk is not processed—neither pasteurized nor homogenized—but it is also more susceptible to bacteria and spoilage. Pasteurization, an important safety measure to reduce spoilage, requires heat that not only kills about 90% of the bacteria but also kills several food enzymes and increases the acid level. You won't find the perfect milk in your grocery store and for very good reason: the shelf life of unpasteurized milk is very short. Unpasteurized milk would almost have to come right out of the nearest cow and you would have to drink it right away—a slight exaggeration but close. When I was living in Austin I purchased some fresh milk at a farmer's market. It was spoiled when I got it home.

Pasteurized milk is good for two to three weeks and is usually delivered to your grocery store from a nearby dairy. Producers of organic milk are few and far between, and their milk can travel long distances to your store. Consequently many of us, particularly those who live in rural America, may only find organic milk that is ultra-pasteurized.

Ultra-pasteurization includes extraordinarily higher heat, pretty much killing everything in the milk and affecting some of the protein such that you cannot make cheese or yogurt with it. The shelf life of ultra-pasteurized milk can be several months if packaged correctly and does not even require refrigeration until it is opened. The organic, ultra-pasteurized milk in the refrigeration section of your grocery is there because you expect it to be, not because it needs to be. So the good news is that ultra-pasteurized milk won't spoil for a long time. The question is, do you really want to drink it?

The bottom line is that there are good reasons to avoid non-organic milk. And there are good reasons to avoid anything ultra-pasteurized. It's your decision. I have chosen to give up milk unless I get lucky and find organic, pasteurized. By the way, while organic, pasteurized milk may not be in the store nearest you, it is less difficult to find organic, pasteurized yogurt—probably because you can't consistently make yogurt with ultra-pasteurized milk.

Use Butter, Not Margarine

As noted above, milk fat (butterfat) is one of the few natural food sources of vitamin D. Manufactured "butter" in the form of margarines is processed, usually includes grain oils, and should be avoided. And in case you need another reason not to eat margarine, some still have hydrogenated oils in them. (You want to avoid hydrogenated oils in anything.)

Here is another issue with butter and milk. A hormone called rbGH or rbST is commonly given to cows to raise their milk production; the consequences of the hormone is another discussion entirely as the FDA insists there is no confirmed health risk to consumers. I do hate to await confirmation of risk. Of course, the perfect butter and milk would be organic from grass-fed cows (that grain thing again) but it might be pricey and hard to find as well. Second choice would be organic, period; milk from cows raised organically will not include rbGH. But unless you are consuming really large quantities of butter, which I doubt, your most cost effective option may be to settle for the ordinary butter. For what its worth, I look for and often find butter from cows not given growth hormones. If you read the labels you will find it.

A few other bits of advice:

- Milk, sour cream, yogurt, and cheese are sources of protein and fat. A serving of each equals a 1-ounce serving of meat/protein. Eat natural cheese. Processed American cheese and Velveeta do not qualify as natural cheese!

- The nutritional value in whole milk, butter, sour cream, yogurt and even natural cheeses is great. However serving sizes matter—large quantities are not required or suggested. The USDA recommends a daily 3-cup equivalent recommendation for dairy, probably because of the calcium included, which amounts to 1.5 servings of protein and over half of the DVA requirement for vitamin B12. Those three cups could include cheese and yogurt. Americans are committed to our milk with cereal and beyond the nutritional value, as I have already suggested, whole milk products are a way to diminish the blood sugar/insulin impact of sweets in all forms, sugar or grain.

- If you are lactose intolerant, then milk is not going to be an option. You will have to get your protein, vitamin B12, and calcium elsewhere. But note that the process of making hard cheeses like cheddar and Parmesan removes the carbohydrate in the milk and thus eliminates the lactose. And even mozzarella has very, very little. Therefore, many of those who are lactose intolerant may still include some cheeses in their diet.

- Yogurt (including Greek yogurt) should only be plain, whole fat and, of course, organic if possible. However, if you are not already a plain yogurt fan, then flavoring may be required. I throw a handful of blueberries on my breakfast yogurt but a dab of honey is also tasty. Flavored yogurt in the grocery is packed with either sugar or high fructose corn syrup. The one exception I have seen with artificial sweetener was, to put it mildly, disgusting.

END NOTES

[1]	Jordan Lite, "Vitamin D deficiency soars in the U.S., study says," Scientific American (March 23, 2009). Online at: http://www. scientificamerican.com/article.cfm?id=vitamin-d-deficiency-united-state (accessed December 17, 2014).

[2]	Of course, the absolute best source of vitamin D is sunshine on your skin, but for a variety of reasons Americans don't get enough sunshine either!

CHAPTER SEVENTEEN

Protein—Meat and Beans

The protein you eat breaks down into amino acids, acids that work full time building and/or repairing every cell in your body. Meat and milk products along with beans are the significant sources of protein. Most common vegetables (not including fruit) also include a small amount of protein. A diet balanced in all of these provides more than enough protein.

The USDA recommends 6 to 8 one-ounce equivalent servings of meat and/ or beans daily for a 2000-calorie diet. This amounts to about 42 to 56 grams of protein. And based on my research, that is a reasonable recommendation on average. There are, of course, varying perspectives on the appropriate amount of dietary protein. For growing teens, adults who do a lot of physical work, and men who are taller and heavier than women, more protein may be required. The more cell building/repairing required, the more protein you need to eat.

The USDA loves to talk about protein in terms of "one-ounce equivalents" and I have used the term already earlier. That can be a bit confusing so let's see if we can clear it up:

- Three ounces of meat or fish is a 3-ounce equivalent. This protein comes "packaged" with fat. Size wise, this is about the size of a deck of cards or a woman's palm.

- An egg is a one-ounce equivalent packaged with fat in the yolk.

- A cup of whole milk or yogurt is a one-ounce equivalent packaged with fat and some carbohydrate. Cream, on the other hand, is only fat.

- A domino-sized chunk of natural hard cheese is a one-ounce equivalent packaged with fat and no carbohydrate. The softer cheeses have a bit of carb.

- Two tablespoons of peanut butter is a one-ounce equivalent packaged with natural fat and some carbohydrate.

- Half cup of the typical beans is a one-ounce equivalent, packaged with a very small amount of fat and a very large amount of carbohydrate starch. So from a protein perspective one cup of beans is equal to 2 ounces of meat.

You can see that it is quite easy to meet your protein requirements without eating a lot of meat. Remember that meat is high in acid and it doesn't take much to meet your B12 requirements. Important, of course, is that the beans be properly treated before eating.

Without considering environmental and humanitarian issues—that is another book—it appears clear nutritionally that wild caught fish and pasture/grass raised beef, pork, and poultry, as well as products like eggs, butter, and fats from these, are better than the alternative. According to the Nutrition Journal, grass-fed beef has significantly higher amounts of omega-3 fatty acids, vitamins, and antioxidants and fewer calories than grain-fed beef.[1] Free-range chickens offer the same value.

Hogs that are pasture raised and eat the naturally available food (including meat, as they are omnivores) are a healthy source of protein. But much of the grocery store pork will have been raised in a feedlot and stuffed with grain just like the beef—with some of the same negative consequences. You can't tell the difference by looking at the package unless it actually says the difference. I choose to have faith in the labeling although many would argue against me.

Unfortunately pasture raised meat is also expensive and sometimes hard to find in any size smaller than half a cow. It is somewhat easier to find wild caught (rather than farm raised) fish, but it may also be expensive. Of course, any meat at the grocery store is expensive. So the guidelines provided below assume that you need to maximize protein while minimizing store-bought feedlot meat. Here are a few carnivorous tips for your protein needs:

- Wild game and lamb, goat, etc., are not typically feedlot raised and are fine sources of Vitamin B12. Venison, bison, turkey, quail, or even squirrels are great options for hunters or people with hunter friends.

- Eat at least two, 3-ounce servings of wild caught (not farm raised) fatty fish (i.e. salmon, tuna, and sardines but there are others) per week. These will make a substantial contribution to your omega-3 needs along with vitamin D and vitamin B12 requirement as well. Canned salmon (preferably red salmon) and tuna will do when fresh is not possible. I should point out that the omega-3 is in the fat, not the meat. So if you throw away the fat, you've missed the point.

- If you cannot afford or bring yourself to eat fish, then the quality of your meat becomes doubly important. You can consider flax or chia seeds in your diet and possibly supplements as well. Flax seed is also an excellent source of fiber but with a high amount of phytic acid.

- In a budget pinch, catch your fish yourself from clean water. Other fresh water, wild caught (not farm raised) fish, while not particularly good sources of omega-3, are still good protein and sources of vitamin B12.

- Most fresh water fish are considered game fish and there are often restrictions on how they can be caught and whether they can be sold. Consequently the fresh water fish you eat in a restaurant will likely be farm raised. For those of us in the American South, this includes the ever-popular catfish. The absolute best choice in a restaurant will be a fish that is advertised as "wild caught."

- The meat in your daily diet does not have to arrive on your plate in large chunks; it doesn't have to be the star player in the meal. Meat in beans for seasoning, meat in vegetable stir-fry, meat in soups and stews, etc., are still meat! Use your imagination.

- Properly prepared legumes (beans and nuts) are excellent sources of nutrition including substantial levels of protein. Vitamin B12 requirements call for some meat, fish, and/or dairy but a good portion of your protein can and should come from plant sources. Legumes are a primary source of protein eaten by vegans and are very cost effective protein alternatives for the rest of us.

- Most peanut butters at the grocery store will include high fructose corn syrup or sugar and extra oil, usually partially hydrogenated. Sorry about that. First look at the "natural" peanut butters. Then pick one that says: "ingredients: peanuts." A bit of salt is probably ok. (You have to be as old as I am to remember how peanut butter used to taste before they started messing with it.) The exciting news is that the number of peanut butter brands labeled as "natural" has multiplied five fold since I began writing this book. More competition means lower prices. Remember that natural peanut butter should be refrigerated after opening. It is the partially hydrogenated oils in non-natural peanut butter that allow you to store it on the shelf in your pantry and you don't want to eat that stuff. One more thing: Bear in mind that peanut butter, as is true with peanut oil, has an omega-6/omega-3 imbalance. A diet heavy in peanut butter is not a good thing but a diet that includes some peanuts can be beneficial except for that small group of people with a peanut allergy. In a perfect world you would soak and roast raw nuts and grind your own peanut or almond butter. Oh, for a perfect world.

- Note: Meat is protein but beans are both protein and starch. A cup of beans for dinner will be two servings of protein, with starch (sugar) in the mix. There is nothing necessarily wrong with this choice unless you have blood sugar problems; just remember that it is two servings (two ounce equivalents) and should be balanced with vegetables. Here again I would bet money that someone you know will eat 4 servings (over a can) or more of beans at a sitting. So if you add 2 to 3 slices of cornbread to the beans—likely because of size to be 4 or more "servings"—you have eaten a lot of starch and, blood sugar is likely to spike. You cannot compensate for that much sugar just by adding a piece of meat. Serving sizes matter and starch is sugar.

- While you should eat the fat on wild-caught fish, remove as much skin and fat as possible from farm raised fish and feedlot, grain-fed meat including poultry because the grain and contaminants ingested by the animal will likely show up in the fat. If the local grocery has only standard commercial meat and is the only source of beef or poultry you have available, all the more reason to keep your beef and chicken consumption to a minimum. Eat more wild caught fish and wild game if possible.

- Where possible, eat fresh meat as opposed to processed stuff like salami, hot dogs, sausage, bologna, canned chili, etc. For one thing, you often cannot know what else is in there besides meat or even what parts of the meat. Read the ingredients on the label. Nitrite preservatives in these products are necessary to keep bacteria at bay but contribute to increased acid levels and inflammation. If you find this to be impossible for budgetary reasons, then lean more toward eggs, cheese, beans, etc. as your primary protein sources.

- A final word on meat preservatives. Preservatives allow food to sit around for a while without spoiling. So you must also know that processed meat without a preservative can't stay in your refrigerator for two weeks like the stuff you are used to. Preservative-free meats should either be eaten/cooked in a couple days or frozen for future use. Read more about this in the next chapter.

- There may be some meat in your current diet, like, say bacon, that you are pretty sure you can't live without and you want it to taste just the way your bacon has always tasted. I confess that bacon is a weakness of mine as well. There is nothing, in my view, better than a bacon, lettuce, and tomato sandwich. And pancakes, at least for me, call for bacon. I suggest that these should be special treats. Bake or microwave your bacon. You won't be able to tell much difference. This, dear reader, is an example of an occasional "treat" that really is a treat.

....

END NOTES

[1] Cynthia Daley, et al., "A review of fatty acid profiles and antioxidant content in grass-fed and grain-fed beef," Nutrition Journal 9 (March 2010). Online at: http://www.ncbi.nlm.nih.gov/pmc/articles/PMC2846864 (accessed December 17, 2014).

CHAPTER EIGHTEEN

Processed Meats

There is meat, and then there is processed meat. The difference seems to matter. Processed meat can be fresh or cured. The products found vacuum packed in a grocery store will be cured, partially or fully cooked, and must contain a preservative, typically sodium nitrite which provides protection against food poisoning and inhibits rancidity in the fat.

Meat processed at home can be fresh (without preservatives) or cured in a fashion somewhat similar to the commercial product and also includes nitrite for preservative. Excessive amounts of nitrite are harmful and the USDA is very specific about the amounts that can be used. Fresh sausage should be cooked within three days, or else frozen. Vacuum packed cured meats can be refrigerated for about two weeks if not opened.

Processed meats, particularly those in the store, usually have a much higher percentage of fat than the meat from which they came. The original fat from the meat is often removed and replaced with pork fat. Sodium nitrite can be replaced with celery juice but that does not eliminate the nitrite. Celery juice can only be a substitute because it is naturally high in nitrates which convert to nitrites and thus accomplish the required preservation. So the store package may say "no nitrites added" but the nitrites are still in there. So, any way you cut it, nitrites it is and will be.

The battle ensues as to the health issues associated with nitrites and I have studied both sides. As is true of fructose and trans-fats, nitrites occur naturally in both meat and vegetables. The issue with processed meats seems to be the amount of nitrites being consumed over and above those occurring naturally in our food and how the nitrite-containing meat is cooked. Studies abound looking for clear relationships between nitrites and cancer, type 2 diabetes, etc. Right now the thing you can find is connections.

But sometimes those connections are really interesting and worth attending to. Studies including almost half million men and women from ten European countries were packaged together and analyzed looking at consumption of red meat, processed meat, and chicken. The goal was to connect the three with the risk of early death. As you probably know, much research is done trying to prove the negative consequences of red meat (pork and beef) consumption; these happen to be the meats most often found in processed meat. The result?

> After correction for measurement error, higher all-cause mortality remained significant only for processed meat (HR = 1.18, 95% CI 1.11 to 1.25, per 50 g/d). We estimated that 3.3% (95% CI 1.5% to 5.0%) of deaths could be prevented if all participants had a processed meat consumption of less than 20 g/day. Significant associations with processed meat intake were observed for cardiovascular diseases, cancer, and 'other causes of death'. The consumption of poultry was not related to all-cause mortality.[1]

Interestingly, the men who had the highest red and processed meat consumption ate the fewest vegetables and fruit. But those who had the highest chicken consumption also had higher intake of vegetables and fruit. I'm still thinking about that one.

A connection is just that. And I must restate that it usually isn't any one thing that threatens your health but rather combinations. We don't yet know why these connections exist and what other factors might have been overlooked. But one thing true of cured processed meat is that it is usually made from red meat (beef or pork), contains nitrites, probably contains more fat, and should be minimized in your diet.

END NOTES

[1]   Sabine Rohrman, et al., "Meat consumption and mortality - results from the European Prospective Investigation into Cancer and Nutrition," BMC Medicine 11 (March 2013). Online at: http://www.biomedcentral.com/1741-7015/11/63 (accessed December 17, 2014).

CHAPTER NINETEEN

Fruits and Vegetables

Your mom's advice to you when you were a kid is as true now as it was then: Eat your fruits and veggies! I'm a mother too so I know she was thinking of nutritional value; we mothers want our children to be healthy. However lots of mothers think all vegetables are alike and that really isn't quite the case. As explained earlier, the sugar in food is called carbohydrate and the differences in vegetables revolved around the amount of sugar predominate in the food.

A review will be worthwhile. Vegetables can be considered in two categories, those with small amounts of simple sugar and those with large amounts of complex sugar. Complex sugar is called starch and any food with lots of starch invariably has lots of calories. Eventually that complex sugar breaks down into lots and lots of simple sugar. For the two thirds of Americans who are weight challenged and all of the diabetics, one danger is in the volume of sugar.

Frequently when I talk about foods that contain predominantly starch, I also talk about table sugar. You saw that in the chapter Grains, Potatoes, and Sugar. If you look up the carbohydrates in plain old granulated sugar you will find only 4 grams in a teaspoon. So why would I have it associated with starches? Perhaps you have guessed the answer already.

If granulated sugar was only delivered by the teaspoon in coffee or tea, you would not have found it grouped together with grains and potatoes. Realistically granulated sugar, fruits, and vegetables have the same kind of sugar configuration — some simple combination of glucose and fructose. But that just isn't how sugar usually arrives on your table. Instead, refined sugar tends to come in cups packed in with the ground-up starch in grain (flour), artistically displayed in the bakery case, on grocery store shelf, or the pie taker on your kitchen counter. That is a lot of sugar.

In other words, volume of sugar really matters, both for your health and your weight. There are lots of foods available to you that have small amounts of sugar and bring amazing amounts of nutrition — as opposed to ground up, refined grain (flour) and granulated sugar which bring no value. Those foods are fruits and vegetables.

The predominant component in that long laundry list of non-starchy vegetables growing in many gardens,[1] is a simple combination of glucose and fructose, along with water, fiber, and a little protein. The value of these vegetables to your health lies less in the frequently miniscule amount of sugar and more in the fiber, vitamins, minerals, and phytonutrients. So you can eat just about all you want of these vegetables with maximum nutritional affect and little impact on your blood sugar or your body fat.

The predominant component in fruit is essentially the same, a simple combination of glucose and fructose, along with water, fiber, and a mountain of nutrients. The difference between fruit and vegetable make-up is this: There is significantly more sugar in fruit and a large component of that sugar is fructose. Some have more fructose than others and, as you learned earlier, glucose raises blood sugar but fructose does not. Just remember that while fructose does not impact your blood sugar, you are not off the hook fat-wise as it is eventually converted to fat by the liver. Over consumption of fructose (in the form of high fructose corn syrup) found in processed food is a danger. But for healthy folk the natural fructose present in two to three servings of fruit daily add a lot of nutritional value and some really nice flavors.

However, just in case you eat an orange (or any other fruit) and it makes you sick, that suggests fructose intolerance. I know people who can't eat oranges or grapefruit. Allergic reactions create inflammation and by some estimates 33% of people have some level of fructose intolerance. If you think this might apply to you, this link lists the total sugar and percent of fructose for a large number of fruits: https://thorfalk.wordpress.com/2011/04/25/healthy-fruits-fructose-edition/. Don't faint when you see that a tomato is actually a fruit.

Eating Your Fruits and Vegetables

With the idea in mind about how important both fruits and vegetables are as "good" carbs, let's take a look at fruit and veggie consumption in our daily diet. Here are some key tips about eating fruits and vegetables:

- The more vegetables the better. There is really no reason to talk about servings of vegetables because you can and should eat as much as you like. But just in case you are interested, a serving of vegetables is 2.8 ounces as defined by the USDA. That is a little bit of cauliflower and a ton of spinach. The spectrum of vitamins, antioxidants, and other nutrients in vegetables is enormous. Eat them.

- If you choose to eat standard grocery store meat (and commercially processed bread), then the vitamins, antioxidants anti-inflammatories, etc., in vegetables and fruits are all the more urgently required in your diet—4 to 6 servings of vegetables per day at a minimum.

- Fruit, on the other hand, should be a bit more restricted. Two to three fruits a day. Fresh fruit is first choice. Second choice is frozen and canned (with no added sugar) is third. Technically a serving of fruit is also 2.8 ounces. Must you carry your scales at all times? In the interest of simplicity this will usually amount to a small to medium solid fruit like an apple and two handfuls of berries. The One Serving of Fruit, Vegetables, Nuts and Seeds website (www.oneserving.com) will be helpful.[2]

- As I said before, however tempting and convenient, fruit juice as a drink is not a good choice. All the fiber is gone and it is the fruit version of "flour"—predigested and hitting the bloodstream full speed ahead. Sugar drinks, of which fruit is one, have more impact on blood sugar than any other food. But if you must drink fruit juice, be sure it really is juice with no added sugar of any kind, make it 4 ounces and even dilute it with water, and serve it with a meal. Juices are best used as flavoring in other dishes. Drink water. Eat the fruit.

- Soft drinks are also sugar drinks and should be avoided—not only for the sugar (which is usually high fructose corn syrup) or sugar substitutes which are sometimes just as bad, but also for the caffeine. Changing to diet drinks does not solve the problem; they are just a different source of trouble. Soft drinks are high acid whether regular or diet. How about water or unsweetened tea?

- Dried fruit has had all the water removed and is thus sugar intensive but still has the fiber. So raisins, craisins, dried apricots, and such are good choices for baking or as throw-on for salads or cereal but not good snacks because of the sugar concentration.

- Vegetables do not include the legume family, beans and nuts or potatoes or rice. They include green, orange, red, white or any other color leafy or crunchy vegetables. Those colors are important as they reflect the particular nutrients in the food. Which is best? There is no such thing as the most nutritious vegetable or fruit. Each and every one brings something important to the table (no pun intended). Before the days of the produce department at your friendly grocery store, people ate the produce that was in season. This would be a good approach, particularly if you have your own garden.

- Grow your own garden or barter with your neighbor. Go to the farmer's market. Learn to freeze or "can" vegetables and fruits for more variety in the off-season or when the budget gets tight.

- As much as possible eat some of your vegetables raw, in salads or by the handful. Digestion—the conversion of carbohydrates into glucose, protein into amino acids, and fat into fatty acids, etc.—takes place with the help of enzymes. Cooking destroys enzymes. Most commercially processed and home cooked foods have had heat applied. Pasteurization of milk and frying food also destroys enzymes. In the interest of safety, eating the typical American meat raw is not recommended, although some people do. So to minimize strain on the liver and pancreas (sources of most enzymes) the more vegetables eaten raw, the better.

- I find The George Mateljan Foundation (www.whfoods.org) to be an excellent source for the specific nutritional value of all vegetables and fruits as well as advice on cooking methods. Take a look.

- The importance of fruits and vegetables cannot be overstated. The nutrients are much needed to help reduce the chronic levels of inflammation so prevalent in Americans today.

END NOTES

1. See the article on "Non Starchy Vegetables," at the American Diabetes Association's website, at: http://www.diabetes.org/food-and-fitness/food/what-can-i-eat/making-healthy-food-choices/non-starchy-vegetables.html (accessed April 12, 2015).

2. "Fruit & Veg.," One Serving of Fruit, Vegetables, Nuts and Seeds website. Online at: http://oneserving.com/category/oneserving/fruit-and-veg/ (accessed February 27, 2014).

CHAPTER TWENTY

A Word
About Fiber

You may remember that if a fat-soluble vitamin is contained in a plant, the fat required to metabolize that vitamin is also included. Remember also that the enzymes required to digest any food are packaged in with the whole food—of course cooking kills the enzymes, but that is another story. Fiber, it seems, is always included in a food requiring it.

Waste that passes out from your intestines is the stuff that did not completely digest as well as a variety of other non-food related elements. Babies whose sole diet is milk, which includes no fiber, are still quite proficient in excreting their waste! Under healthy circumstances the amount of waste left over from animal food digestion is passed from the body along with the fiber inherent in the carbohydrates we also eat.

This brings us to a common issue with constipation found among the American population. Medications, inadequate consumption of water, and lack of exercise are certainly contributors to constipation, but a very central issue is the lack of fiber in the diet. We got in trouble on fiber at about the same time that we began consuming large quantities of refined grains (from which most of the fiber had been removed) and stopped consuming vegetables (which have significant fiber as well). Note that while the enzymes are killed when vegetables and fruit are cooked, the fiber is still there. And while the minerals in untreated whole grain are locked up, the fiber is still there and available.

When your diet converts to whole grain, limits grain servings, and begins to include an appropriate amount of fruits and vegetables, any fiber deficiency you might have is likely to disappear. Normally the answer to a fiber deficit is eating whole foods that contain fiber, not special fiber supplements or laxatives. However, as in everything else, things are not always normal. So if diet doesn't do it for you and you are otherwise drinking enough water and staying active, then you may need to see your doctor.

CHAPTER TWENTY-ONE

Read the Label

So far on our journey together you've gotten one piece of advice from me over and over: Read the label! The Food & Drug Administration requires prepared and packaged foods to be labeled for their ingredients and nutritional value.[1] Use that to your advantage. Get in the habit of checking out what food companies are actually putting in the stuff you are buying—and then use that knowledge to make good choices. Here are some tips that I think are important when it comes to reading the label:

- <u>Always</u> read the ingredients on the label of a processed food before buying.

- Beyond the stuff I have already mentioned, generally speaking a long list of ingredients means the food is more processed. That's bad. A long list of words you can't pronounce is worse still!

- As a reminder, pay close attention to the Total Carbohydrate information because it can fool you. As I write this I am looking at that info on a box of pasta. Here's what it says: For one ½ cup serving (not much) the…

  - Total Carbohydrates are 46g (which is a lot)

  - Dietary Fiber is 4g

  - Sugars are less than 1g.

  Despite the fact that the label says less than 1g of sugar, the net effective sugar after subtracting the fiber in this pasta is actually 42g because the carbs are starch ground into flour.

- Bonnie Taub-Dix's Read It Before You Eat It and other similar books can help enormously in understanding food labels including additives and supplements.[2] Ms. Taub-Dix credits the Center for Science in the Public Interest website for some of her information.[3] She points out, "Just by looking at a list, you might not know that caseinate, whey solids, and lactalbumin are all derived from cow's milk, or that hydrolyzed vegetable protein comes from wheat, peanuts, soybeans, and other legumes."[4] Indeed! As we've already seen, foods like wheat, peanuts, and soybeans are prime sources of food allergies, and "hydrolyzed vegetable protein" is actually MSG.

• Speaking of MSG, it's worth making a point about it separately. MSG is a food additive that is supposed to enhance taste. It isn't good for you though, and it should be avoided. Many people are sensitive to MSG, and what's worse, it can be hard to identify because it hides out under many different names in processed food. Deanne Repich, the founder and director of the National Institute of Anxiety and Stress, Inc., has written about the connection between MSG consumption and anxiety symptoms.[5] She notes that the following food ingredients will always contain MSG:

- Monosodium glutamate
- Calcium caseinate
- Textured protein
- Monopotassium glutamate
- Glutamate
- Glutamic acid
- Gelatin
- Sodium caseinate
- Yeast nutrient
- Autolyzed yeast
- Hydrolyzed corn gluten
- Hydrolyzed soy protein
- Hydrolyzed wheat protein
- Hydrolyzed protein such as vegetable protein

In fact, according to Ms. Repich, if a product label says it contains any form of 'hydrolyzed' protein then you can bet that it contains MSG.[6]

• Finally, in his book, Fast Food Nation: The Dark Side of the All-American Diet, Eric Schlosser dazzled me with information about food additives, specifically flavorings.[7] It turns out that the taste and smell of bananas, citrus, just about anything, can be added to processed foods. And those additions are simply nothing but chemicals that you will never identify on the label because the label will say either "natural" or "artificial" flavorings. Both of those will still be created or extracted chemicals. The commercial flavorings business is huge. So remember the Pop-Tart that I mentioned much earlier in the book? It smells and tastes like the fruit because they added chemicals. The more processed food you eat the more unidentified chemicals you are consuming. And if you happen to have digestive issues these additives could well be contributing. Read the label!

....

END NOTES

[1]   See "Labeling & Nutrition," U.S. Food & Drug Administration website. Online at: http://www.fda.gov/Food/IngredientsPackagingLabeling/LabelingNutrition/default.htm (accessed January 6, 2015).

[2]   Bonnie Taub-Dix, Read It Before You Eat It: How to Decode Food Labels and Make the Healthiest Choice Every Time (New York: Plume, 2010).

[3]   In particular, see this page: http://www.cspinet.org/reports/chemcuisine.htm (accessed December 17, 2014).

[4]   Ibid.

[5]   Deanne Repich, "Could MSG Sensitivity Affect You?" Articles Factory website (May 1, 2006). Online at: http://www.articlesfactory.com/articles/health/could-msg-sensitivity-affect-you.html (accessed December 17, 2014).

[6]   Repich, "Could MSG Sensitivity Affect You?"

[7]   Eric Schlosser, Fast Food Nation: The Dark Side of the All-American Meal, Reprint edition (New York: Mariner Books, 2012).

CHAPTER TWENTY-TWO

Special Notes

Now I'd like to offer some special notes on a few items that seem to be of interest to many people these days: organic foods, hardboiled eggs, fresh and frozen foods, and storing whole grain foods.

Organic or Not Organic?

Organic means that the plant seed was not genetically modified (GMO) plus the environment/soil within which the food was grown or the food fed to the animal was not subjected to chemical fertilizers or pesticides. The perfect food is not only organic but also grown locally. Because perfect organic food from a grocery store is typically more expensive, the next best option is food grown locally. Thus go for the local garden, either your own or at a farmer's market. There are often local farmers who grow organically but can't afford to invest in the regulatory approvals required to label their product as "organic." But perhaps neither organic nor local is possible.

If you have a choice, vegetables and fruit usually eaten peeled are the best non-organic choices. For example, an organic avocado or orange may not be worth the price because of the nice, thick skin. But, and this is important, you should wash these well. There will be contaminants on the skin. This is particularly critical if you are zesting the fruit to include in a recipe or if you plan to put a slice of lemon in tea or on a plate.

Going one step further, we often eat the skin of products like potatoes and apples and this is really a good thing as much of the nutrition and fiber is in the skin. Thus organic, or at least local, would be best. As suggested earlier, eating the vegetables and fruit is important, organic or not. Just be sure to wash vegetables and fruit carefully before eating them.

Hardboiled Eggs

Eggs, especially free range eggs, are a super food. They're a source of protein, B12, omega-3, and good fat that also works very effectively to help slow down blood sugar. Thus, there is real value in using them for a variety of applications—including snacks. Eggs are one of those foods whose reputation has gone back and forth. Researchers are now convinced that they are a good food with lots of benefits. So eat up!

It is the peeling of the hardboiled egg that can be a challenge. I have researched and tried just about every method of peeling hardboiled eggs only to have one method work great one day and the same method fail miserably another day—no matter how I cook them. Happily I now know the problem revolves around the age of the eggs.

The eggs you find in the grocery store have been in cold storage for several weeks if not months—they peel easily. The fresh, free-range eggs you buy from your neighbor are brand new and they are very reluctant to let go of the shell, nature's way of protecting the chick that might be growing. A peeled egg that looks like it has been used for target practice is fine for mashing into egg salad but won't make a pretty deviled egg.

Perhaps you know how to tell if an egg has gone bad by placing it in water. A spoiled egg will float and a fresh egg will lay flat on the bottom of the container. As an egg ages it begins to tilt in the water. Let a dozen fresh eggs sit on the shelf in your fridge for two or three weeks and they will begin to tilt and should peel just as well as the ones from the grocery store. I shared this epiphany with my egg lady, Penny, expecting her to be impressed. She said, "Didn't I tell you that? You always have to let fresh eggs sit for a couple weeks before hard boiling them."

Fresh vs. Frozen

Beyond the organic discussion, freshness is the most important thing with vegetables. So, of course, the perfect vegetable is one you plucked from the garden this morning and cooked this afternoon. The frozen vegetables at the supermarket are typically flash frozen right after harvest and the nutrition is "locked in" so they are close to fresh. But the vegetables in the produce section of the grocery store were usually picked long ago and have likely deteriorated nutritionally.

Frozen vegetables don't lend themselves to salads or anything else calling for raw but they are just fine when used as ingredients in a cooked recipe. For example, I have used frozen vegetables in both chili and beans and could not tell any difference. So if you have freezer space take advantage of good buys on frozen onions, peppers, peas, green beans, or any other vegetable, particularly if the vegetable is out of season and not available in your garden.

Sometimes the amount of perfect vegetables coming out of your garden (or your neighbor's, or mother's) this morning is in excess of what you can cook today or tomorrow. So what to do with them? In a few months there won't be any tomatoes or squash (or anything else) growing in your garden. But you still have to eat! There are two possible answers. You can freeze your own or you can "can" them like my grandma did.

My grandma's cellar was well lined with canned food so they never ran out regardless of the season. But, of course, grandma didn't have a freezer. So she had no other option. Canning is a great alternative but if you are not ready to become a "canner" because the equipment is too expensive or you just don't have the time, then consider freezing your excess vegetables and fruit instead. Your county extension office and the Internet can all provide direction on freezing.

Storing Whole Grain

Here is an interesting bit of information. Back in the old days—say in Robert E. Lee's time, when refrigerators weren't available—there was a problem with milled whole grains going bad. The culprits in the spoilage were the oils in the bran and (particularly) the germ. These are the two parts that happen to contain most of the nutrition. So over time, especially as commercial bread became common, the bran and germ were eliminated and refined flour absent the most nutritious parts became the norm.

A whole grain is protected by the hull, and the protection is lifted when the hull is removed and the grain is ground up. Refined flour is nothing but the endosperm and there really isn't much there needing protection so it can sit on the shelf at the store or your pantry for a very long time. At least until the weevils find it.

A whole grain flour and a home-made whole grain bread will be susceptible to spoiling. This includes stoneground corn, which isn't whole grain if it is "de-germinated" because they removed the germ. Keep the grain tightly sealed in your freezer and buy only the amount you will use in a short period of time. If the only reason you have flour is to batter a chicken or make cornbread, you might consider just using white, unbleached flour and de-germinated cornmeal. It will be much easier to store.

CHAPTER TWENTY-THREE

An Evolution vs. a Revolution

Despite all the reasons for making the lifestyle changes I've identified so far, there are some that really are more important than others. In order of priority, the top three are:

1. First, as odd as it may seem, your primary goal is to control blood sugar. That's true whether you are diabetic or not. This is largely accomplished by managing the amount of starch and sugar in your diet. You can help yourself towards this goal in a number of ways:

    a. Manage your grain and potato consumption to a maximum of two servings per meal, six servings per day of the appropriate serving size. Maybe you will make these be whole grain, soaked or sourdough, and maybe not. But keeping to that limit will also minimize the nutrition loss from phytic acid in whole grain and achieve a significant reduction in your consumption of omega-6.

    b. Always balance starches and sugars in every meal with protein and fat, along with fiber in fruits and vegetables.

    c. Try to eliminate refined sugar, white or brown, and anything containing high fructose corn syrup. Do your sweetening with natural sources like fruit or even honey.

    d. Eat as many servings of vegetables a day as you can work in. Potatoes and rice are starches, not vegetables.

2. Second and not far behind is increasing your consumption of omega-3

and decreasing omega-6. If you are a typical American, your grain consumption is likely out of whack. So taking steps to curb it in concrete ways is important:

    a.   Throw away all of your grocery store oils except EVOO and a small bottle of canola. Grain oils are a huge source of omega-6. Store the canola in the refrigerator.

    b.   Eat two servings of wild caught coldwater fish like salmon, tuna, or sardines per week. If necessary these can be canned.

    c.   Make your meat be wild caught fish and free range meat (including wild) as much as you can. If this is not possible, then broaden your protein options. A lot of meat is not really required. Remember that you can substitute eggs, cheese, yogurt, and milk to get protein. You can also add beans and nuts of all sorts to your diet (making sure to soak and cook/roast them properly in order to maximize the nutrition and digestibility).

    d.   Note that the grain priority above also fits into this category, because of the omega-3/omega-6 implications of eating grain-based foods.

3.   Minimizing your purchase and consumption of commercially processed food. I could go into great detail on this one, but in reality my priority #1 pretty much takes care of that for you. For sure, the stuff you don't want to eat is hiding out in those boxes, bags, and other kinds of containers. If it comes in a vacuum-sealed plastic bag, it probably isn't good for you.

So what does this look like at mealtime? It can look lots of different ways. And it doesn't mean that you are going to have to do food gymnastics every time you sit down to eat. Here are some simple examples of easy meals that may not be perfect but are balanced:

•   A ham sandwich with whole grain bread and chips is a perfectly acceptable meal. Just add cheese, lettuce, tomatoes, and whatever or include a small side salad or some chopped vegetables. Make that one serving of chips, no more than 15 or so. Add an apple or other piece of fruit. Even if the meat in this sandwich includes preservatives and the cheese is made from ordinary cow's milk, you will still have kept blood sugar under control and maximized nutrition.

- A hardboiled egg, a slice of cheese, sliced vegetables, a pickle, three or four crackers, and a handful of properly prepared nuts.

- A grilled cheese or egg salad sandwich with whole grain bread, sliced vegetables and ranch dip. A piece of fruit for your sweet tooth.

- Half peanut butter (natural) sandwich or peanut butter with a few whole grain crackers, or peanut butter on apple slices. ½ cup of yogurt with a dab of honey and a handful of berries.

- ½ cup of homemade bean dip (chickpeas or any other bean properly prepared) with vegetables for dipping. Hummus is really nothing but a bean dip. A piece of fruit.

Please make your store bought bread the best possible. No trans-fats, sugar or high fructose corn syrup, or bad oils. But if you get trapped into whole grain with soybean oil, all the more reason to limit the amount of bread in your diet. From a blood sugar management perspective, the central issue is how much bread (refined or whole grain) you eat, particularly at one sitting. Again, in an honest assessment of blood sugar, cornbread is a combination of ground corn and ground wheat, whether the grains are whole grain or not. Frequency and serving size (about 2X2 inches) are the important issue in the world of managing blood sugar.

There is no good reason I can think of that would require the use of the grain oils like corn, soybean, etc. Buy the EVOO (and the canola if necessary), toss out whatever else you have in the pantry (it's probably rancid anyway), and store the canola in the refrigerator. As I mentioned earlier, the best EVOO is "first cold pressed" (which means no heat is applied and the least effort was required to remove the oil) and is probably organic but if you can't find or afford that, then settle for the EVOO you find on the shelf at the grocery store. Or you might look at TJMaxx or HomeGoods where I discovered it much easier to find cold pressed and the discounted prices are not far out of line with the grocery store.

Let's talk potatoes. Anyone who eats in a restaurant knows that potatoes, usually fried and in large quantities, are staples. They are high starch and can easily impact blood sugar. This means that a monster baked potato, big stand-alone bowl of potato soup—with lots of potatoes—or a plate piled high with

French fries can be a blood sugar problem. But a cup of potato soup along with a protein, and salad of some sort is a well-balanced meal, a small to medium baked potato with butter and/or sour cream, broccoli or another vegetable, etc., along with some meat is also balanced. (By the way, whenever possible leave the skin on a potato and eat it. Nutrition and most of the fiber is in the skin!) The central issue is the amount of potato. If you can control portion sizes, there is no reason why an occasional meal balanced with protein, vegetables, and fruit cannot include potatoes. This is an excellent example of the importance of making the food taste really good. Make those potatoes a treat rather than just something else on the plate.

Unless you can afford to buy lots of wild caught fish and non-feedlot animals, you absolutely have to make beans, eggs, cheese, and such regular parts of your daily diet. Operating on the "treat" theory espoused several times above, use meat the way many Europeans do. You don't have it very often but when you do, make it a happy source of conversation for days to come.

If the meat is that important to you, then start looking around for a local source of free-range meat. It isn't impossible but may be a challenge. Nonetheless, you can eat store bought, feedlot meat, just keep it to a minimum and be sure to remove the skin and as much fat as possible. Bear in mind that the majority of the fat in poultry is usually on the outside under the skin and easily removed. The fat in beef is on the outside and also in the "marbling" of the meat. Despite your best efforts, you will consume more fat eating equivalent amounts beef than chicken. What I call "feedlot" ground beef should be purchased as lean as possible. Use a little olive oil if more fat is needed. And, for sure, don't forget that the accompanying vegetables are providing the natural antioxidant helping to counteract the negatives of the feedlot meat.

I want to point out that you can find free-range chickens and their resulting eggs somewhere locally. Such eggs are easily available in my tiny county so I doubt yours will be an exception. In fact, in many towns people are returning to the old practice of raising chickens in their backyards—which means they get fresh eggs daily! For the financially challenged, eggs (along with beans) are an excellent, cost effective standby for protein.

You also don't have to go to a specialty store in a big city to find cheese from grass-fed cows. You are, in fact, more likely to find these from local producers. Admitting that it comes from Ireland, I buy Kerrygold at Sam's Club. But again, while you may be eating lots of eggs, a serving of cheese is pretty small. So unless cheese is your primary source of protein, a regular cheese is probably okay.

Finally, the best early control of serving sizes is to fill the plates from the stove and take them to the table; don't tempt yourself with a bowl full of mashed potatoes, a pile of fried chicken, a basket full of bread, or a bag of chips.

In other words, you don't have to go full bore into the Almost Perfect Diet. Rather there are a few selected things that are the highest priority. Your first step is to attend to those. As time progresses and you see how well you, your family, and your budget feel, you can advance your evolution even further. But in the event that you never go one step further, you are still much better off than you were before.

The eating habits of children, however, may be a challenge all its own. You trained them well, so pick your fights. All the following could also apply to the bigger "children" in your family. My dad, who was otherwise perfect, would often say, "Do as I say, not as I do." That didn't work well for him and it probably won't work well for you.

What you'll read in the next chapter is just one approach for children. But there are many parents who are dealing with healthy diets for children so see what others are doing. I cheerfully refer you to 100 Days of Real Food (www.100daysofrealfood.com), a website created and maintained by Lisa Leake.[1] Lisa's following grows every day and you will love her ideas as her whole program revolves around the needs of children. You will be exposed to literally hundreds of recipes and the experiences of many walking in your same footsteps. Her site and her advice can be a great resource!

....

END NOTES

[1]   Lisa Leake, 100 Days of Real Food website. Online at: http://www.100daysofrealfood.com/ (accessed December 17, 2014).

CHAPTER TWENTY-FOUR

For the Children

This is not a weight loss program, but for those children who have become carbohydrate dependent and are paying the price in their size, weight loss could be inevitable. I encourage you simply to strive to gain control of your children's diets and let the weight take care of itself. The exception would be the child that has actually become obese; in that case, you'd need the help of medical and dietary experts.

Step one is to explain to your kids what is going to happen and why, especially if they are old enough to understand. "First we are going to do this, and then we are going to do that." And remember, they probably won't like it at first—so try not to weaken.

Recently a friend of mine was discussing this book with other friends within the earshot of her six year-old grandson. When Charlotte said, "Ms. Pat says that we should get our sugar in fruit," her grandson piped up, "Well, that's not going to work for me." You should expect resistance from older children and be happy if your youngsters are still young enough to start out right!

Eliminate soft drinks as daily fare. Dispose of what you have and don't keep any more in the house. Everyone needs to drink water or, as an alternative, milk or unsweetened tea. If you feel it necessary, add soft drinks to the weekly treat list. If necessary, put juices on the treat list or designate two days a week as juice days. Dilute real apple juice (no sugar added) with water and provide it with breakfast two days a week. An apple can be served as a daily snack but apple juice should be served with a balanced meal.

Next, accomplish an all-at-once conversion to the best possible bread, crackers, and cereal. Then control the number and size of servings by what you serve or have available in the house. Don't turn your child loose to fill a cereal bowl. Fill it yourself or, if she is old enough, show how to measure the right amount by using a measuring cup. Encouragement and applause are good things.

Choices are also a good thing. Here is one idea. Go to the grocery store alone and pick out four whole grain cereals you find acceptable, if you can find four. Bring home all four and let everybody taste test with the appropriate milk, berries or other fruit, and a few nuts, of course. Do the same thing with crackers. Then the children can choose which one(s) they want.

Post a list of acceptable snacks on the refrigerator for everyone to see. And do away with anything in your pantry that doesn't fit the bill. This is particularly important if your children are at home by themselves; as you well know, they will eat what they want if it is there and available. At this point, don't fret over what they eat at friend's houses unless they eat all their meals there, which is a different problem. If this becomes a real issue long term, you may have to figure something else out.

For snack time, try the following:

- Cut oranges into slices, bag and store them in the refrigerator for easy access. Or use mandarins or clementines if the children can be convinced to peel. I didn't know that peeling would be such a big deal until I helped prepare a lunch for 4th graders at a school event. Cutting oranges into slices solved the problem and they were all eaten.

- Keep a bowl of fruit on the kitchen counter.

- Bag up some nuts for quick servings.

- Slice vegetables (whichever ones you think will be accepted most readily) and store them in the refrigerator for easy access. Have the dip ready if needed.

- Slice some cheese, hard boil some eggs. Put a few slices of leftover meat in a bag.

When somebody (children or you) wants something to eat quickly, such as after school, the above could be their choices. A child authorized to wield a knife might put peanut butter on apple slices or possibly even a few whole grain crackers. That said, I encourage you to do everything possible in the beginning to limit daily grain servings to meals, especially if you will not be there to supervise.

My experience and that of many others is that children are much more willing to try something new if they took part in the preparation. My friend Amy, a 4H coordinator, tells me that children involved in school gardens are always willing to try and more likely to actually like the vegetables they harvest from their garden.

With your children (and maybe yourself or your spouse) create a list of weekly "treats." Just because the stuff we crave isn't particularly good for us doesn't mean that the craving will go away quickly. Sugar and salt are truly addictive. What is it that they really want to eat but isn't on the daily list? This might be chocolate chip cookies, PopTarts (heaven forbid), brownies, Doritos, potato chips, ice cream, or a soft drink. Maybe little Mary actually wanted those cookies from the store that had all that bad stuff in them, but you could just bake up your own homemade version with the good stuff instead. And never allow more than one serving of the treat—that means "a" cookie, not a sack of cookies or a half can of soda pop, not a whole bottle.

Once a week each person (including you) is allowed to select from and eat a treat. Make it a special event, a party if you will or the "we do treats on Wednesday nights," but allow them to decide when it will be. Over time the choices of weekly treats will become shorter as children (and adults) will lose interest in stuff that won't, eventually, taste nearly as good as they remember it. I can personally attest to this. However, some things may be on the list forever—cookies, brownie, ice cream, and other sweets—preferably homemade with healthy ingredients. Homemade ice cream for a family picnic is a wonderful treat but is less exciting if ice cream gets eaten daily.

Growing children need to eat. Your goal is to manage what they eat. You will work a miracle when you get control of grain and sugar consumption. If they want two eggs, fine. If they want two oranges, fine. If they want to snack on crackers or cookies or Fritos or potato chips, probably not fine.

I regret to tell you that the food in the school cafeteria probably isn't going to fit your standard; a lot of starches will be served. You can either treat this as a meal eaten at a "friend's" or you can provide a lunch to take to school. (Lisa Leake does very creative work with school lunches on her website— www.100daysofrealfood.com.)

I do realize that it is a lot easier to stock the pantry with a variety of chips, cereal, cookies, Twinkies, and bread and to fill the freezer with stuff to jam in the oven or microwave. Convenience has gotten us all in trouble. Cooking time is rarely the issue with a meal; rather the preparation time before cooking is the problem. So do the prep earlier. That makes the cleanup after the meal a lot easier as well.

Tomorrow's casserole, soup, or chili can be prepared today or yesterday, at your convenience, and stored in the refrigerator until cooking time. Tomorrow's salad can be chopped today, stored and sealed, for tomorrow's use. Vegetables intended for roasting can be parboiled and stored until roasting time and parboiled vegetables will roast much faster. But I can tell you from experience that parboiling really isn't necessary if you prepare your vegetables and put them in the oven to roast while you make the rest of the meal.

Success will require some planning. Maximize preparation by having meals that will provide for other meals. For example:

- Boil or roast a chicken for one meal and then use the leftovers to make chicken enchiladas or pizza, put atop or into a salad, for lunch sandwiches, or for snacks. Same is true for any meat.

- Make a big casserole or pot of chili and freeze half for another time. Freeze half of that roast or chicken and thaw it out later for another meal or snacks.

- A big pot of soup can cover lunch on another day or be warmed up for an after school snack.

- A pot of beans used at one meal can become refried beans, be added into a soup or a salad, or even frozen for another day.

- Consider what you have frozen and work that into your menu. Remove from the freezer the evening before and let it thaw in the refrigerator.

- Tonight's dinner can be cooking all day in a crock pot even if you are gone the whole time. Consider your and your family's schedule(s) for the week and make one or more of those busy nights include a crock pot dinner. My granddaughter benefits greatly from her crockpot because her family not only has dinner ready to go but the leftovers also go to work with her husband for lunch the next day. Some say that dried beans don't cook well in a crock pot, although canned beans do, but even that is worth a try. Check the Internet for recipes. Just about anything else you can think of short of pizza can be made in a crock pot.

Finally, and this may be really tough, stay out of fast food restaurants. Keep your refrigerator stocked with a variety of acceptable foods and pack a meal if necessary in order to get to the baseball game on time. If you allow your children to break all the rules in a restaurant, they will never cooperate at home. That said, there could certainly be a local eatery with whole grain bread, good meat, vegetables or salads, etc.

I pray for your encouragement and at least a modicum of cooperation on the part of your family. You will ultimately be happy with the results.

CHAPTER TWENTY-FIVE

The Smolder Becomes a Flame

We've talked at some length about the causes of inflammation and how it affects health, but you may not have connected every one of those dots. If not, you may still not fully understand the consequences of a bad diet. In this final chapter, I want to provide a few summaries of some of the most common diseases.

Osteoporosis: Cause and Effect

Osteoporosis means porous bones. Uncorrected, the bones eventually cannot support the weight of the body. When that happens, they begin to fracture. Bone loss is usually greatest in the hips, spine, and ribs. Nearly one third of those who sustain an osteoporotic hip fracture enter a nursing home within one year. And one in five of those will die within that year.

The bones are the calcium, magnesium, and phosphorous alkaline mineral reserve of the body. You may remember these as the minerals locked up in phytic acid in whole grain, beans, and nuts. The absence of bone calcium is generally accepted as the reason for increased bone fractures, but American consumption of typical calcium sources like milk or calcium supplements doesn't seem to make the problem go away. According to Susan E. Brown, author of Better Bones, Better Body, low bone density in other populations in the world doesn't seem to result in more fractures, and countries whose populations consume the most calcium also seem to have the highest osteoporosis rates.[1]

Calcium is the most common mineral in the body and 99% of the calcium in the body is in bones and teeth. The 1% balance is in the blood and very tightly controlled by the body in order to maintain the blood's pH level. When the blood acid level starts to go up because the diet hasn't provided the alkaline ash (calcium) needed to neutralize acid, the body calls on the bones to send calcium.

Over time, this is supposed to be a healthy process. The bones give up a little calcium and then build it back up. However, if the amount of acid remains excessive in the diet/lifestyle, then the body won't have the nutrients needed to replace the calcium. Thus bones can become osteoporotic. Not consuming enough calcium, vitamin D, and magnesium plus depletion of existing bone mineral are the primary causes of osteoporosis.

Calcium is found in milk and vegetables and even in meat if the meat is raw or minimally cooked. However, even if enough calcium is eaten, the absence of vitamin D and magnesium in the body will prevent calcium absorption. Vitamin D can be found in fortified milk, eggs, and butter along with fish— all foods containing cholesterol. However, vitamin D is primarily synthesized by the cholesterol in our skin in contact with sunlight. Magnesium (primarily found in whole grains, beans, and vegetables) is required for that conversion of sunlight to vitamin D.

The intake of calcium in the American diet exceeds that of almost all other countries so the absence of calcium in our diets isn't likely to be the cause of our calcium deficiency. Rather, according to the Scientific American, three-quarters of teens and adults in America are vitamin D deficient.[2] And most American diets are deficient in magnesium. Several factors could be involved. For one, Americans (sadly including children and teens) have become more sedentary, sitting at a computer or in front of the TV as opposed to working or playing outside. Further, concerns about skin cancer make the use of sunscreens prevalent. Sunscreen blocks the UVB rays required for vitamin D synthesis. Exercise and some exposure to the sun are important to bone health. Also, many of the foods that are likely to naturally include vitamin D are those sometimes discouraged such as eggs and butter.

Dark green, leafy vegetables as well as other vegetables, legumes (beans, nuts, and seeds) along with whole grains are the major sources of magnesium.

Americans consistently fail to eat the needed amounts of daily vegetables. Further the grains, beans, nuts, and seeds most commonly eaten are untreated and thus the magnesium is locked away in phytic acid.

In summary:

- Failure to eat the foods that provide calcium, magnesium, or phosphorus will cause depletion of bone minerals.

- Chronic body acidosis (inflammation) caused by failure to balance acid in the diet along with excess sodium, coffee and colas with caffeine, and tobacco and drugs also contributes to bone mineral depletion.

- Finally, failure to exercise and spend enough time in the sun prevents the body from making vitamin D which is required for the body to absorb calcium.

Obviously eating the diet outlined in this book, including whole milk, eggs, butter, and fish is critical. However, getting outside in the midday sun, arms uncovered and without sunscreen for 15 to 30 minutes per-day, is the absolute best solution for adequate Vitamin D. For exposure longer than 30 minutes, use sunscreen. The exposure provided in the spring and summer of temperate climates is expected to provide enough stored vitamin D for the winter months. If this is not possible because of weather or season, then it is all the more urgent to reduce acid levels in the body through diet. And a consultation with your doctor may suggest taking a vitamin D3 supplement.

Despite doing all the "right" things, an aging body sometimes fails to metabolize all the nutrients properly. My own experience is relevant.

Bone density tests over several years found me to have "osteopenia," the precursor to osteoporosis, despite the fact that I spend a lot of time in the sun. My doctor prescribed and I took Fosamax for some time to no avail. Finally I grew concerned about the advertised negatives of this and other similar drugs and elected to stop taking it. Instead the doctor and I agreed to add a substantial vitamin D3 supplement. Sure enough, in the next test my bones had returned to normal.

Obesity and Type 2 Diabetes: Cause and Effect

None of us really needs a definition of overweight or obese. We know it when we see it, a third of Americans are overweight and another third are obese. We see them often —maybe in our own mirror. So how do we get that way?

Our bodies use protein, fat, vitamins, and minerals to keep our parts in working order but our energy comes primarily from carbohydrate sugar (glucose). Any excess energy is turned to body fat. A car runs on petroleum fuel but, unlike humans, the gas tank has a maximum capacity. Our human fat cells, sometimes to our detriment, can hold an almost unlimited amount of fuel. In fact, if necessary, we can even add more fat cells. Most overweight conditions are due to our diet but not necessarily for the reasons we may think.

Your body will convert body fat to energy when necessary. But if you get all your energy from the carbohydrates in your diet, particularly processed, refined foods, body fat conversion is not necessary and fat will simply accumulate. Over 60 percent of Americans, including most diabetics, are carrying a good amount of fat padding, frequently in the form of visceral fat strapped around our mid section.

Those carbohydrates are present in the blood in the form of blood glucose. The conversion of blood glucose into energy requires the hormone insulin which is manufactured by the pancreas. Diabetes is a condition where insulin is not doing its job and there is too much glucose (sugar) hanging around in the blood. The percentage of the American population that is or is destined to become diabetic is skyrocketing.

The Centers for Disease Control & Prevention (CDC) estimates that 3.7% of people aged 20–44, 13.7% of people aged 35 – 64, and 26.9% of people over 65 have diagnosed and undiagnosed diabetes. Further, between 2005 and 2008 35% of U.S. adults aged 20 years or older and 50% of those aged 65 years or older were pre-diabetic.[3] Consider for just a minute what a huge portion of the population this represents.

The CDC defines pre-diabetes as individuals whose blood glucose after an overnight fast or hemoglobin A1c levels are higher than normal but not yet classified as diabetic. Diagnosed diabetes in the United States more than tripled between 1980 and 2011.[4] And the 60 % of overweight or obese Americans with substantial amounts of visceral fat are at particular risk.

Eating the typical American diet, the older and heavier you get the greater the chance that you will become diabetic. Cardiovascular disease is the cause of about 33% of the deaths in the US but that same condition will be the cause of death for over 65% of diabetics.[5] Do the math. This is not a good direction.

Type 1 diabetes (juvenile diabetes) exists when the pancreas is damaged and fails to secrete insulin. Type 2 diabetes—originally called "adult onset," but now children also have it—exists when the body has an increasing need for insulin because the body cells are insulin resistant. While insulin resistance and deterioration of insulin supply can be the result of genetics (my dad had diabetes), predisposition is not a guarantee of diabetes. The sad American diet seems to be the enabler. It is complicated.

There are two other uncommon forms of diabetes not associated with diet. One is a slow-developing autoimmune diabetes called LADA (or "Latent Autoimmune Diabetes of Adults") and the other form is MODY (or "Maturity Onset Diabetes of the Young").[6] MODY actually includes several different conditions depending on which gene(s) are out of whack. About 80% of diabetics are overweight or obese but still 20% are not.[7] Some of the thin diabetics find themselves to have one of the more rare diabetic forms. I am one of the 20% but I am happy to report that I am an ordinary type 2 diabetic.

It is this kind of diagnostic complexity that requires that a doctor be involved in your diagnosis and treatment. Nonetheless, regardless of the cause, part of the treatment plan for every single form of diabetes includes the same sort of dietary discipline discussed in this book.

So overweight or not, type 2 diabetes will usually start with excess consumption of processed refined starches (grain and potatoes) and sugar. And for sure, once type 2 diabetes starts to develop—likely years before the doctor identifies diabetes—fixing the diet is the best chance to ward it off. Further, once we become diabetic, controlling sugar and starchy carbohydrate consumption becomes the most crucial element in managing the condition. Medication may or may not be required but America is full of diabetics with heart disease, missing body parts, and kidney failures who think that taking medicine is all they have to do. They are wrong. Medicine alone is not going to prevent blood sugar spikes.

Carbohydrate consumption that causes no problem for non-diabetics can create high blood sugar for diabetics and pre-diabetics whether they take medication or not. Fat that has accumulated over the years isn't going anywhere as long as blood sugar remains out of control. Diet management then becomes crucial.

Not long ago I ran into a diabetic friend I hadn't seen in some time. She has been obese as long as I have known her so I was amazed to see how much weight she had lost. She was glad to tell me how she did it. Seems she had been to a nutritionist who told her to do two important things—limit her daily starch carbohydrate consumption to a specific number and always include a protein when she eats those carbs. She had lost 36 pounds so far and was celebrating. Her words to me were, "I wish somebody had told me this sooner." The good news is that you don't have to be diabetic to lose weight using that same strategy.

A blood measurement known as A1c shows how much blood sugar is "glycated" or stuck to your hemoglobin (red blood cells) as an indication of your average blood sugar over a three- month period. A normal A1c would be between 4 and 6%. However, reducing A1c average blood sugar alone may not be enough. Blood sugar highs along with blood sugar lows might average quite well but still leave you in danger. The walls of your blood vessels and your pancreas aren't watching the average.

As we saw in the chapter Blood Sugar and Insulin, persistently high blood sugar and/or blood sugar spikes along with the consequent insulin can still damage the blood vessels and result in "long-term irreversible vascular and connective-tissue changes. These changes include diabetes ... specific complications such as retinopathy, nephropathy and neuropathy and ... atherosclerosis; potentially resulting in heart disease, stroke and peripheral vascular disease."[8] This is the stuff that causes blindness, amputations, and heart attacks.

Again, type 2 diabetes does not just show up on a random Thursday. Rather, it creeps up slowly over time along with a few or a bunch of extra pounds. As a result of my research I found myself to be diabetic and, while I had gained about 15 pounds over many years, I have never been overweight. My genetics were inescapable—almost everyone in my father's family was diabetic and all except one were reasonably slender. When I went back through many years of blood lab results (I keep everything forever), I could see that my fasting blood sugar (the measure you get when you haven't eaten for 12 hours) had been creeping steadily up while generally remaining within the "normal" range.

Was I diabetic or not? I wanted to know. So I found an amazing web site (www. phlaunt.com) created by Jenny Ruhl, a MODY diabetic, and got directions on how to test myself.[9] I bought a meter and test strips and followed those directions, which amounted to eating a plain boiled potato and then measuring my blood sugar at 1, 2, and 3 hours. Sure enough, those "postprandial" (meaning measured after eating) measurements were not good. So I contacted my doctor and found myself diabetic.

Fortunately I am able to manage my diabetes solely with diet—which means I monitor my starchy carbohydrate and sugar consumption carefully and measure my postprandial (is that not a great word?) blood sugar regularly. In time I found that I could stay within the parameters of normal blood sugar if I eliminated starches entirely. Another diabetic friend once told me she wanted to keep all her fingers and toes and be able to see them for a very long time. I totally agree and make sure my diet matches that interest. My risk tolerance is very low. And I should mention that I have lost that extra 15 pounds which shows how easily weight can be lost if carbohydrate consumption is controlled.

Genetic predisposition (it runs in the family) is a factor but avoidance is often possible. I think I might have prevented my condition had I just known what was important sooner. I shudder to think what those skillets of American fried potatoes and bread I ate as a teen would do to my blood sugar today even though I would just love to be able to eat them again.

Minimizing your chances of type 2 diabetes and obesity starts with management of insulin demand as a normal part of your diet. The guidelines in this book will help avoid blood sugar spikes—the sources of insulin demand—and also prevent fat accumulation. However once pre-diabetic or diabetic you may not be able to eat as much or perhaps any starches or sugar as they will drive spikes.

So how can you know if you have a potential problem? Those of you who never go to the doctor may not get a clue if you don't take steps on your own. Those of you who go to the doctor annually are asked to fast (not eat anything) for 12 hours before blood work. The blood work will check your fasting glucose

(FPG) level and the doctor will typically decide if diabetes is a concern based on that number. In my case that number was still within the normal range.

If the number is out of range the doctor would then check your A1c level to see how much blood sugar is stuck or "glycated" to your red blood cells. And perhaps a two-hour glucose tolerance test within which you will drink a bottle of glucose (sugar water) and your blood sugar will then be checked hourly. This accomplishes somewhat the same thing as eating the potato referred to earlier.

As I mentioned earlier, A1c is reflective of an average and does not show how far your sugar goes up or down after meals. So it is possible to have an acceptable A1c level (below 6), which I did, and still have an issue with your blood sugar. Only the two-hour glucose tolerance test identified my diabetes. The pattern is the only clue; a higher number every time you test suggests that insulin resistance and deficiency is building. But, of course, I didn't know that.

On the day of my two-hour glucose tolerance test my fasting blood sugar was 91, well within the normal range. In the glucose tolerance test, normal glucose tolerance will show glucose not rising above 140. A condition called impaired glucose tolerance (IGT) will show a rise to between 140 and 199.[10] I went from 91 to 247 in one hour and fell only to 179 at two hours before finally plummeting to 67 at three hours. They call this diabetes and it had been developing for a very long time.

About two years before my diabetes was discovered I began having tingling in my feet, neuropathy which I now know is fairly common in diabetics and can spread upward, become painful, and eventually become serious. I discussed this with my nephrologist (the wrong doctor by the way) and he asked if I had diabetes. Of course I said "no."

So now you can see the danger. Diabetes creeps up on you. Years before diabetes becomes obvious, vascular disease development can start. Injured vessels can result in kidney damage (nephropathy), nerve damage (neuropathy), retina damage (retinopathy) and, of course, cardiovascular disease. According to the National Diabetes Information Clearinghouse (NDIC), diabetes is the leading cause of kidney failure, non-traumatic lower-limb amputations, and new cases of blindness among adults in the United States—all due to damage in the vascular system.[11] Smoking also causes the same sort of damage and thus diabetic smokers are doubly at risk.

Of course when you can't see, or your feet hurt, or you have a heart attack you will go see a doctor who will hopefully find the diabetes. But at that point, you are in recovery as opposed to prevention.

If diabetes is found with extreme blood sugar the doctor may prescribe insulin to achieve some immediate control of blood sugar. But in most cases he/she can first suggest diet change and exercise. Most Americans never accomplish either, even if the doctor sends them to a nutritionist as mine did. Failing that, the doctor will prescribe one of several medications depending on analysis of your situation. There are medications that reduce the amount of glucose being released from the liver (glycogen), stimulate the pancreas to release more insulin, slow the absorption of carbohydrates, enhance insulin sensitivity in body cells, and/or combinations of several.[12] Note that none of those medications will prevent a blood sugar spike.

In the end, most doctors monitor diabetic conditions using the fasting blood glucose level and regular checks of A1c. Most diabetics I know go home with their medication and then eat whatever they want with not-so-good results. According to the American Association of Clinical Endocrinologists (AACE) this helps explain why in the year 1994 only 44% of patients achieved an A1c level of less than 7% and then by the year 2000 this proportion actually decreased to 37%.[13] "Normal" A1c is 4-6%.

You can manage your A1c only by managing postprandial blood sugar, described earlier as managing insulin demand. Again according to the AACE and The American Diabetes Association (ADA),[14] blood sugar targets for diabetics should be:

- A1c less than 6.5%

- Fasting plasma glucose less than 110 mg/dL

- 2 hour postprandial plasma glucose less than 140 mg/dL

These would be artificial and not-normal blood sugar goals in diabetics intended, it appears, to avoid periods of low blood sugar. Low blood sugar (hypoglycemia) can be life threatening as can extremely high blood sugar. The dangers of middle of the road but still abnormal blood sugars take longer to get you, but get you they will. A person with normal blood sugar metabolism would rarely ever have a postprandial blood sugar over 110, an a1c above 5.5, or fasting blood sugar above 95. My goal was and is normal blood sugar.

The question is, how does one get to "normal?"

In the beginning I tested a lot of different combinations of foods to see what would happen to my blood sugar. Understanding the need to slow down the sugar digestion I thought I could figure out how much protein and fat I would need to eat with my carbs so that I could still eat starches. Actually I just wanted those carbs to just disappear because I really didn't want to give up potatoes and bread. I'm sorry to say that it just did not work and I eventually found that absolute tight control of my blood sugar could only be achieved if I gave up all starches. Of course Dr. Shallenberger in his book the Type 2 Diabetes Breakthrough[15]and Dr. Bernstein in his book Dr. Bernstein's Diabetes Solution: The Complete Guide to Achieving Normal Blood Sugars[16] had already told me all of this, but I was praying to be an exception.

Type 2 diabetes is a self-managed disease. For the vast majority of us, what, when, and how much we eat is the number one driving factor in blood sugar. Please learn from my experience. If your diet has been poor by the terms discussed in this book, diabetes/heart disease runs in your family, or you start developing neuropathy, then you are at risk. First fix your diet and then go get checked out by your doctor. The earlier you catch your problem the less damage you will do to yourself. Be prepared to do just as I did. Test different combinations of food until you find out what you can eat and still keep your postprandial blood sugar well below 140. Your doctor can determine medication requirements based on your success.

Fair warning! In the beginning you will use at least eight test strips per day measuring and recording blood sugar when you arise in the morning, before each meal and then after, and before you go to bed. I often used even more, taking postprandial measures at 1 hour and then 2 hours. But you aren't measuring for fun; you will be adjusting what you allow yourself to eat until you see what diet will achieve a good result. This shouldn't take more than a few weeks.

I suggest you use a test meter and strips that can be purchased off the shelf at the pharmacy. My own primary care doctor explained to me that not many doctors will write you a prescription for so many test strips primarily because insurance and Medicare won't pay for them. Once you figure out what you absolutely cannot eat or how much of some things you can eat, then you just follow your rules and fall back to fasting measurement and a random measurement during the day just to make sure things aren't changing or to find out how much damage you did with that slice of chocolate cake or gourmet bread.

As mentioned above, hypoglycemia is low blood sugar and is usually the outcome of a excessive insulin medication or a blood sugar high such as reflected in my personal glucose tolerance test. Because I never allow my sugar to be high I am not troubled with bouts of hypoglycemia but you may be. Your nutritionist can give you guidance. But if you have no nutritionist, then ask Jenny Ruhl on her website (www.phlaunt.com). Having said all this, do your best to have a doctor and a nutritionist, but also take responsibility for your own body.

Not long ago I asked another diabetic with not-so-good (at least in my opinion) fasting blood sugar and A1c if he was measuring after meals and recording what he was eating. He said "no." Being the pushy sort, I wondered why and was told, quite firmly, that the doctor had not told him to. The goal is protect your health, not to have someone else to blame when it goes bad.

Allow me to close with the story of my friend Julia. She has been diabetic for many years with high cholesterol and triglycerides, and was born with only one kidney. She has always had trouble achieving control of her a1c, fasting, and postprandial blood sugar despite exercising and taking her medication faithfully, truly eating a much better diet than most diabetics. She has also always been plagued with fatigue and couldn't get rid of about 30 extra pounds. I finally convinced her to try giving up starches, particularly grains, just as a trial. In two weeks her fasting blood sugar and postprandial sugar were straightening out, she had lost 7 pounds and, most exciting of all, was full of energy every day. This could be you.

Atherosclerosis: Cause and Effect

The transportation system for the nutrients, water, and oxygen in our bodies is the cardiovascular system, often referred to as the bloodstream, including the heart, arteries, veins, and capillaries. When the blood fails to flow, nothing else matters. While there are a number of points of potential failure, one of major importance is the buildup of plaque in the walls of arteries causing partial or complete blockage of the stream itself, a condition commonly called atherosclerosis. That buildup is concurrent with chronic inflammation.

Along with obesity and diabetes, smoking is one of the leading causes of cardiovascular disease in the United States. According to the American Heart Association, smokers are at a greater risk of developing atherosclerosis, which can lead to heart attack, coronary heart disease, and stroke. In the case of smoking, the chemicals in the cigarettes cause inflammation and the ultimate build-up of fatty substances in the arteries.

According to the United States Environmental Protection Agency, the prevalence rate of heart disease and stroke remained constant between 1997 and 2009 while the death rate actually declined, presumably because the total number of inpatient cardiovascular operations and procedures increased by 33% between 1996 and 2006.[17] Still, the death rate from cardiovascular disease was about one in every three deaths in 2006.

Current strategies and treatments appear to be reducing the CVD death rate but the increase in obesity and diabetes discussed earlier suggests that prevalence rates may soon be on the upswing. The American Heart Association forecasts that by 2030, unless something changes, 40.5% of the US population is projected to have some form of CVD and medical costs will have tripled.[18] According to the Center for Disease Control and Prevention, during the past 30 years the prevalence of obesity in children 6 to 11 years has increased from about 4% to more than 20%.[19]

Fat, cholesterol, and other substances do, indeed, build up in the walls of arteries and form hard structures called plaque when inflammation of the artery walls allows for it. And according to all we've learned so far, apparently inflamed walls are allowing for that quite a lot.

If you have atherosclerosis you should be under a physician's care. But part of your treatment has to be preventing further damage. Do all you can to eliminate sources of inflammation in your body. The first steps are exactly the same as those for obesity and diabetes—follow the guidelines in this book. Get control of your weight and blood sugar.

....

END NOTES

[1]   Susan E. Brown, "Rethinking osteoporosis: Halting bone loss and reducing osteoporosis risk," Better Bones website. Online at: http://www.betterbones.com/osteoporosis/default.aspx (accessed February 27, 2014).

[2]   Jordan Lite, "Vitamin D deficiency soars in the U.S., study says," Scientific American (March 23, 2009). Online at: http://www.scientificamerican.com/article.cfm?id=vitamin-d-deficiency-united-state (accessed December 17, 2014).

[3]   Figures listed are for 2011. For the most up-to-date statistics, see Centers for Disease Control & Prevention, "2014 National Diabetes Statistics Report," CDC.gov. Online at: http://www.cdc.gov/diabetes/data/statistics/2014StatisticsReport.html (accessed January 7, 2015).

[4]   Centers for Disease Control & Prevention, "CDC Number (in Millions) of Civilian,

Noninstitutionalized Persons with Diagnosed Diabetes, United States, 1980–2011," CDC.gov. Online at: http://www.cdc.gov/diabetes/statistics/prev/national/figpersons.htm (accessed February 27, 2014).

[5]   American Heart Association, "Cardiovascular Disease and Diabetes," AHA website (heart.org). Online at: http://www.heart.org/HEARTORG/Conditions/Diabetes/WhyDiabetesMatters/Cardiovascular-Disease-Diabetes_UCM_313865_Article.jsp (accessed February 27, 2014).

[6]   Jenny Ruhl, "MODY: A Rare Form of 'Type 1.5' That is Often Misdiagnosed," Blood Sugar 101 website. Online at: http://www.phlaunt.com/diabetes/14047009.php (accessed December 17, 2014).

7   U.S. Department of Health & Human Services, "Do You Know Some of the Health Risks of Being Overweight?" Weight Control Information Network website. Online at: http://win.niddk.nih.gov/publications/health_risks.htm(accessed December 17, 2014).

8   Julie Hatfield, "REVIEW: Advanced Glycation End-products (AGEs) in Hyperglycemic Patients," Journal of Young Investigators (October 2005). Online at: http://www.jyi.org/research/re.php?id=575 (accessed January 7, 2015).

9   Jenny Ruhl, "Am I Diabetic? How to Test Your Blood Sugar To Find Out," Blood Sugar 101 website. Online at: http://www.phlaunt.com/diabetes/14046889.php (accessed December 17, 2014).

10   David M. Nathan, et al., "Impaired Fasting Glucose and Impaired Glucose Tolerance," Diabetes Care 30:3 (March 2007).Online at: http://care.diabetesjournals.org/content/30/3/753.full (accessed February 27, 2014).

11   See "National Diabetes Statistics Report, 2014," by the Center for Disease Control & Prevention. Online at: http://www.cdc.gov/diabetes/pubs/statsreport14/national-diabetes-report-web.pdf (accessed January 7, 2015).

12   "Oral Diabetes Medications Summary Chart," Joslin Diabetes Center website (joslin.org). Online at: http://www.joslin.org/info/oral_diabetes_medications_summary_chart.html (accessed February 22, 2014).

13   Harold E. Lebovitz, et al., "ACE/AACE Position Statement," Endocrine Practice 12:1 (Jan/Feb 2006). Online at: https://www.aace.com/files/positionstatement.pdf (accessed February 22, 2014).

14   Nathan, et al., "Impaired Fasting Glucose and Impaired Glucose Tolerance."

15   Frank Shallenberger, The Type 2 Diabetes Breakthrough (Laguna Beach, Basic Health Publications Inc., 2005).

16   Richard K. Bernstein, Dr. Bernstein's Diabetes Solution: The Complete Guide to Achieving Normal Blood Sugars, Fourth edition (revised and updated) (New York, Little, Brown & Co., 2011).

17 "Cardiovascular Disease Prevalence and Mortality," U.S. Environmental Protection Agency. Online at: http://cfpub. epa.gov/eroe/index.cfm?fuseaction=detail.viewInd&lv=list. listByWhereYouLive&r=216637&subtop=381 (accessed February 22, 2014).

18 Paul Heidenreich, et al., "Forecasting the Future of Cardiovascular Disease in the United States: A Policy Statement from the American Heart Association," Circulation (March 2011): 933-944. Online at: http://circ. ahajournals.org/content/123/8/933.long (accessed February 27, 2014).

19 Centers for Disease Control & Prevention, "Childhood Obesity Facts" CDC.gov. Online at: http://www.cdc.gov/healthyyouth/obesity/facts.htm (accessed February 27, 2014).

CHAPTER TWENTY-SIX

In the End, a New Beginning

Yesterday I stood in the hall outside a meeting room listening to Helen describe (complain) about her indigestion. I tried to explain gently to her why she should consider changing her diet. Perhaps you think that it was none of my business, but I see it differently. Isn't that what friends are for? Unfortunately for her, that change is rather urgently needed due to her health and also very inconvenient for her lifestyle. Both of her parents had heart trouble, her father was a diabetic, and she is very overweight. Because we are friends and she knows I am writing this book, she listened. (Well, at least she got that I'm listening look on her face but her eyes were saying something different.) "Just consider it," I said. She assured me she would but my confidence is not high. Maybe this book will help.

There are three major factors involved in our health—our genetics, our environment, and our food. Our genes are passed down generation to generation. Those genes determine our height, distribution of fat, intelligence, hair or eye color, and heaven knows what else. In some cases those genetics will also present us with a health condition no matter what we do, but in other cases we inherit only a propensity for a health problem—a problem that we can ward off by how we live our lives. Your genes are what they are. But you do have control of how you live your life.

Everything we put in our mouth and swallow, or breathe in, or even absorb through our skin can have a positive or negative effect on our health. I could have written a lot about the chemicals in women's makeup, hair treatments, and skin care. Chemicals in fertilizers, pesticides, herbicides, or fungicides can be dangerous when absorbed into our food or through our skin and collected in our soil and water. And a lot could be said about over-the-counter drugs, prescription medications, and of course "social" or recreational drugs. These are all potential health dangers as well as, in some cases, treatments for health conditions. But the one health hazard that impacts every living, breathing person every day is the food he or she eats.

Truth is, there is nothing simple about the relationship between your diet and your health. As you can probably tell by this point, even a limited understanding requires more interest and attention than most can muster (and certainly more than is possible in a hallway conversation). Our culture is inexorably attached to food, and this is not a new condition! A thousand years ago was exactly the same. The only difference lies in the food itself and the knowledge about it. Our ancestors likely knew next to nothing about how their bodies used the food they ate. They didn't have to know, because there was nothing else to eat but the natural food in the animal and plant life of their environments. But your situation is different.

Over three years of serious research were required for me to write this book. I started in one place and ended up somewhere entirely different. All that time the rest of you were living your life, going to work or digging in your garden, raising children, maybe writing your own book, and eating whatever tasted good and was easy to fix. You didn't have time to invest years learning about something that you shouldn't even have to know. But if you have reached this chapter in the book, you now know you may need a new beginning.

Nobody wants to spend his or her life counting calories, studying the pros and cons for a particular food, or analyzing the nutritional value and possible penalties attached to the meal about to be eaten. And most of us don't have to. If you believe that the knowledge you have gained from and the guidelines provided in Its All About the Food are right, you can just shove amino acids, omega-3/6 fatty acids, cholesterol, triglycerides, free radicals, vitamins, and calories to the far reaches of your mind. You can join your ancestors eating the natural meat and plants in reasonable proportions without a second thought.

But for a few of you, the basic rules for a healthy, balanced diet will still leave you with an unhappy digestive system or migraine headaches, as examples. You found yourself in the chapter on Enzyme Deficiencies, Autoimmune

Diseases, and Allergies. So your new beginning will first require you to work a little harder figuring out what in this "well-balanced diet" doesn't work for you and adjust your diet accordingly. Take the extra steps however time consuming and aggravating they are. Use this book as a resource, and use the medical, nutritional, and spiritual resources available to help you as well.

Attend to your diet. Attend to your life! All of our lives can be simpler, more comfortable, and perhaps even somewhat longer. They can certainly be healthier—in body, mind, and spirit. If you have embraced that idea and found it to be true, then congratulations! You are no doubt now living in a way that is more healthy, happy, and whole.

About the Author

Pat Smith is a retired corporate executive known for her ability to analyze and fix problems. She has served as chairman of Ouachita Village Inc., a non-profit organization in Montgomery County, Arkansas, focused on the food and nutrition needs of the surrounding community. She is dedicated to helping people make positive, healthy choices about food and nutrition.